Hair, Headwear, and
Orthodox Jewish Women

Hair, Headwear, and Orthodox Jewish Women

Kallah's Choice

Amy K. Milligan

LEXINGTON BOOKS
Lanham • Boulder • New York • London

Published by Lexington Books
An imprint of The Rowman & Littlefield Publishing Group, Inc.
4501 Forbes Boulevard, Suite 200, Lanham, Maryland 20706
www.rowman.com

16 Carlisle Street, London W1D 3BT, United Kingdom

British Library Cataloguing in Publication Information Available

Library of Congress Cataloging-in-Publication Data

Milligan, Amy K., 1982- author.
Hair, headwear, and Orthodox Jewish women : Kallah's choice / Amy K. Milligan.
p. cm.
Includes bibliographical references and index.
ISBN 978-0-7391-8365-6 (cloth : alk. paper) – ISBN 978-0-7391-8366-3 (ebook)
1. Hair–Religious aspects–Judaism. 2. Jewish women–Religious life. 3. Jewish women–Conduct of
life. 4. Modesty–Religious aspects–Judaism. I. Title.
BM726.M56 2014
391.5088'296832--dc23
2014029919

Printed in the United States of America

For Ele, z"l
Truly, a grandmother has never been more cherished.

* * *

רַעְיָתִי יָפָה הַנָּךְ
יָפָה הַנָּךְ
נֵיסוֹי עֵינַיִךְ
לְצַמָּתֵךְ מִבַּעַד
הָעִזִּים עֶדֶר כִּעֲרֶשׁ
גִּלְעָד מֵהַר שׁוּגָּלְשֶׁ

How beautiful you are, my love, how very beautiful! Your eyes are doves behind your veil. Your hair is like a flock of goats, moving down the slopes of Gilead.
—Song of Songs 4:1

Contents

Acknowledgments

As an elementary school student one of my favorite "hobbies" was going to the library to work on book reports. These were self-assigned projects: I would peruse the card catalog to find topical books and write up a report of my "findings." One afternoon, I was diligently taking notes on different methods of paper recycling when my mother was approached by a classmate's mother. The woman was distraught. She had no idea that we had an assignment due at school. My mother was forced to sheepishly admit that I was doing book reports for fun. To this day she still worries that the other woman assumed that I was being coerced into my "research." It was with the same sense of enthusiastic learning that I embarked upon the crafting of this study. Along the way there are many who have helped and aided me in the process.

I am incredibly lucky to have a close and loving family. My husband, Heiner Kessler, followed me across the world so that I could pursue my dreams. His kind spirit, joyful heart, and keen wit are an inspiration. My parents, Dan and Kathy Milligan, did not fear an intellectually curious child and modeled a love of learning and compassion for others. Now, as we face my father's increasingly debilitating health problems, the strength, humor, and love of my family overwhelms me. Some of my earliest childhood memories are of standing on a chair next to the stove while I cooked with my grandmother, Eleanor Stroud (z"l). She taught me to take joy in cooking, travel, animals, and family. Her strength, ability to care for others, and resiliency of spirit continue to inspire me. I would be remiss if I did not also mention my two canine family members, Brandi and Darcy, who faithfully sat by my feet while I crafted this text.

The mentorship of Simon Bronner has been profoundly instrumental in my life. As I struggled as an interdisciplinarian to find my place in the world of academia, Simon took a chance on me and my research, something for which I will forever be grateful. I am appreciative of his constant guidance, incredible work ethic, honest critique, and wry sense of humor.

I am also indebted to Christina Bucher, Charles Kupfer, and Andrea Lieber, who have provided me with support and feedback throughout the process. Additionally, Louise Hyder-Darlington and the Elizabethtown College High Library staff worked tirelessly to help me locate resources. I am thankful for the support of friends and colleagues, including: Susan Asbury, Teresa Berger, Sally Clark, Andy Dunlap, Jennifer Dutch, Heather Kanenberg, Andrea Legnini, Carly Miller-Carbaugh, Sue Ortmann, Arline Rochkind, Steve Scott (z"l), Matthew Singer, Amy Shorner-Johnson, and Evan Smith. I am also indebted to the rabbinic knowledge of Rabbi Leah Berkowitz—who always knows the perfect balance between being a best friend and discussing *halakha*.

Finally, this study would not have been possible without the cooperation, interest, and support of the members of Degel Israel Synagogue. They have allowed me into their lives, encouraging me to ask questions, and challenging me to think outside of myself. In particular, I am grateful for the guidance of Rabbi Shaya Sackett and his wife, Buci Sackett. They helped to pave the way for my inquiries. For all of the women who made space for me at their tables, opening both their hearts and homes to me, I am eternally grateful. Thank you for entrusting me with your stories. I have done my best to retell them with love and respect.

Prologue

This study is an ethnographic inquiry into the lives of Orthodox Jewish women in a small nonmetropolitan congregation. My study varies from other congregational studies or Jewish ethnographies in two primary ways: it brings the often overlooked stories of Orthodox women to the forefront, and it probes questions as to how their location in a small community affects their behavioral choices, particularly regarding the traditional practice of hair covering. This practice is unique to women's traditions and points out the importance of examining the women, not just because they are often overlooked in congregational studies, but also because their cultural role may be marginalized in studies as a result of their lack of a central role in worship. My study questions their contribution to Orthodoxy as well as their concept of their Jewish identity in a nonmetropolitan setting.

This investigation concentrates on women and Jews as subjects in comparison broadly to the dominant American Christian society and locally to the unusual mix of other pietistic groups such as the Amish, the Mennonites, and the conservative Brethren of Lancaster County, Pennsylvania. The entry point of hair study is important religiously among pietistic groups, but it is often neglected as a symbolic system among ethnographers because of the demise of what I call "hat culture" in American society. Many religious groups use hair as a "significant symbol," as social psychologist George Herbert Mead identifies the kind of objects that in social interaction have a special representational role in mediating communication and identity. In this study, significant symbols form an association between the self and God in addition to society. My treatment of hair works toward explaining its rich and deep symbolism, particularly for Orthodox women.

Hair, whether we show it or not, forms part of our self-identity. How we choose to style, display, color, tease, shave, or cover it demonstrates and communicates our perception of self and can, at times, represent community allegiance. Still, hair is so familiar that it is often overlooked. As the most organic form of self-expressed fashion, it is easy to forget that hair warrants separate study. Each morning we make decisions about how to style our hair—or as my husband reminds me, lack of hair—to convey how we wish others to perceive us or how we feel about ourselves. Included in this is the choice to cover hair or the head in order to make a profound statement about identity and religious and/or cultural values.

I also see an intrinsic connection between hair covering and headwear. That is to say, although hats function as part of clothing studies and hair is traditionally considered bodylore, in my approach the two are intertwined. The ways in which individuals consider their hair, as well as the ways in which they conceal or reveal it, are comingled in such a way that I believe it impossible to fully separate the two. This study probes the choice of Jewish women to cover their hair or their heads with the understanding that there are motivations that exist both within and outside of the women's awareness. I hypothesize that their situated context in a small community informs the women's motivations to help negotiate the tensions of living in a nonmetropolitan area, while at the same time meeting their desire to have a feminized Jewish ritual.

Although women are at the center of this ethnography, it is not an exploration of the feminism of Orthodox Jewish women. Rather, I probe issues of religious traditionalism without the assumption that traditionalism equals disempowerment of women. I question the meaning women find in tradition and consider the motivations they have for engaging in traditional behavior. If men are free to engage in ritualized behavior without it positively or negatively affecting their masculinity, why do studies of women presume anxieties of femininity? I wrestle with the women's viewpoint that they consider themselves most valued and validated in traditional contexts.

Equally important is the focus on the role of women in the survival of American Orthodoxy, particularly in a small congregational setting. Many aspects of traditional behavior—keeping a kosher kitchen, for example—are not public. Because of this, the female role in the maintenance of religious tradition often goes unrecognized. Hair covering, which I argue has a profound impact on the women who engage in the practice, is an externalization of these private practices and is perceived as symbolic both for the wearer as well as for viewers. The title of this work, "Kallah's Choice," reflects the significance of this decision. A *kallah*, or bride, makes the decision as to whether or not she will cover her hair after marriage. In doing so, she externally announces her level of religious observance, in particular her commitment to maintaining an observant Jewish home.

Approaching these questions as a religionist and American Studies scholar has allowed me to pull from a rich array of scholarship, including folklore, theology, psychology, and ethnography. Bringing these tools to bear on my subject, I find from a variety of angles that Jewish hair covering, although a traditional behavior stemming from a religion steeped in patriarchy, has been used by some women as a tool of empowerment.[1] It is through this practice that the women of Degel Israel Synagogue indicate to themselves, to other Jews, and to the larger local community that they are committed to living an observant lifestyle. They have beat the odds and are continuing to survive as a small community of Orthodox Jews on the periphery of American Judaism—a feat that can be largely credited to the hard work and innovative spirit of the women of the congregation who are as imaginative with their hair covering choices as they are with solutions to other issues facing their community.

Throughout this study, my role in the community of Degel Israel Synagogue has been one of "personal stranger," a vantage familiar in American ethnographic literature.[2] That is to say, I have functioned as a participant observer while at the same time forming relationships with members of the synagogue. My role as an ethnographer has not been limited to sitting on the sidelines. As an outsider coming into the community, especially as one who was interested in analyzing their choices and practices, there was a certain degree of objective distance that I maintained. However, at the same time, my experiences at Degel Israel have been deeply personal. Time spent at worship was not in observation but active participation. Likewise, outside of worship, I ate in the homes of members, drove older members to doctor's appointments, attended university lectures together, and shopped for clothing, food, and, of course, hair coverings with various women. I also answered as many questions about myself as I asked the women. Most commonly they were interested in my research, shared acquaintances, and my family life. Privately I was asked about my own spirituality and whether or not I considered myself a feminist. These questions always were asked respectfully and helped to form comfortable and honest relationships.

I was able to integrate into the community fairly quickly, which was largely aided by my familiarity with Jewish culture. The congregation is open to hosting inquisitive guests, but integration into synagogue life is made much easier when one has Hebrew skills, an affinity for familiar traditional foods like gefilte fish, and an understanding of and respect for the Orthodox lifestyle choices and Jewish law. Still, the individual members of the congregation are the real reason that I was able to integrate so easily into their community, as they invited me to join them at dinner tables filled with laughter, stories, and tales of heartache. Indeed, the life of an ethnographer is always an adventure.

In this study, I have made a conscious effort to include the women's stories and voices alongside of my analysis. This research, at its core, cannot be removed from its context. These are genuine women with real experiences. To remove their voices would take the heart out of my work. As part of the informed consent process, all of the women were aware that their stories were part of a research project that would be shared with the larger community and ultimately published. Still, I have chosen to change their names and certain identifying details. I have elected to do so because their names are not relevant to the study, and I have represented their viewpoints without revealing their identities.

Some literature within progressive Judaism as well as by non-Jews suggests that, seen through the lens of "modernism," Orthodox Jews are intellectually or culturally backward. It is my sincere hope that in reading the stories of the women of Degel Israel Synagogue, as well as in my detailed analysis of their approaches to the Jewish tradition of hair covering, that readers will appreciate the complexity of traditions with which Orthodox women engage and the self-consciousness with which they intellectualize the practice of these traditions. The story of these women, interwoven with a congregational and ethnographic study, paints a picture of what it means to be a contemporary Orthodox Jew surviving on the fringes of both the local and religious community. It is not an easy life, but one that they have proven adept in navigating despite what many would consider insurmountable odds.

NOTES

1. I understand patriarchy to be an issue both in American society and culture as well as within the Orthodox Jewish community. Within Orthodox Judaism, patriarchy functions in terms of issues like only male ordination, the roles that women are allowed within synagogue life, the expectation of traditional gender roles, and the limited active voice that women are afforded in religious dialogue. I contend that although outsiders are quick to label Orthodox Jewish women as oppressed, they execute power and agency within the religious community in often unrecognized ways.

2. See Michael Agar, *The Professional Stranger: An Informal Introduction to Ethnography* (New York: Emerald Group, 1996); Elliot Liebow, *Tally's Corner: A Study of Negro Streetcorner Men* (Lanham, MD: Rowman and Littlefield, 1967); Elliot Liebow, *Tell Them Who I Am: The Lives of Homeless Women* (New York: Penguin, 1995).

Chapter One

A Hairy Subject

Approaches to Hair and Hair Covering

Tyra Banks had carefully selected new hair styles for each of the models she sought to mold into "America's Next Top Model." The fourteenth cycle of models commenced their journey on this popular reality television show with a drastic makeover.[1] At Sally Hershberger's famous salon, Brenda cried in anguish as her red hair was cropped short. Raina's hair emerged with darker hue to enhance her sex appeal. Naduah's hair, however, posed the most significant problem. Having shaved her head as a sign of independence from the tight-knit religious circle in which she was raised, only her eyebrows could be groomed by the hair stylists. Her fellow contestants marveled at how she appeared like an alien and very exotic with her newly bleached brows. Tyra Banks proclaimed that the participants were no longer just pretty girls—they had morphed into models. Their changed hair styles marked the beginning of their journey on the show. For the contestants of *America's Next Top Model*, their hair initiated a transformation into the world of high fashion.

Indeed, hair is transformative for many individuals. Women, in particular, are targeted by the media and advertisers who use cultural pressures to draw attention to their hair. Because American culture assumes that a woman should have long hair, women are faced with abundant choices as to how to style their hair—which extends to greater symbolic attention than men. Whether it is shampooing, combing, styling, brushing bangs out of the eyes, flipping the hair over the shoulder, or covering their hair, women constantly engage their hair as part of self-expression. It serves as an external display of how a woman wishes to be perceived, how society or culture encodes her, and of her taste, personality, or convictions. In fast paced contemporary

America, merely glancing at a woman's hairstyle allows us to classify her: the long blonde free-hanging hair of a young singer; the impeccable bun at the nape of the neck of a military officer; the practical soccer-mom cut; the slouchy pony tail of a college athlete; the professional office-friendly bob. Many Americans can recognize the heart shaped covering worn over the tightly bound hair of Amish women and are familiar with Muslim women's *hijab*.[2] They are, however, less *au fait* with the traditional head covering practices of Jewish women. Observers might recognize *payot* (sidelocks) or *yarmulkes* (Yiddish, the traditionally male Jewish skullcap; also known as *kippot* from the Hebrew)[3] on Orthodox men, but there is a general lack of awareness of Jewish female hair covering—a practice which is crucial to the social dynamics of Orthodox women.

In this chapter, I begin by clarifying my approach to hair covering and establish the roadmap for the following chapters. The culmination of this chapter is an introduction to my hybrid methodology, which approaches hair as an inclusive symbol, marker, and object that is used as part of ritualized behavior. In this approach, I demonstrate the importance of hair study in a congregational context as an entry point into understanding Orthodox women, their roles, and the ways in which small town Orthodox women beat the odds and survive in otherwise arid soil.

APPROACHING HAIR COVERING

Although Islamic hair covering practices received attention in recent years, and scholars of "Plain" (Anabaptist and Pietistic) Christianity and Revivalist Christianity discuss head coverings, relatively little academic research has been produced concerning the practice of hair covering found within Orthodox Judaism. Scholars have generally overlooked hair covering, discussing its use only in passing, not taking time to address its motivations and psychological implications for Orthodoxy. Such treatment renders hair secondary in religious dialogue, limiting it to the realms of religiously mandated dress or as ritualized behavior.

My analysis of contemporary hair covering practices is an extension of an ethnographic study of Degel Israel Synagogue, located in Lancaster, Pennsylvania. I discuss the context for this study in chapter two, "Covering Jewish Women: The Congregational Context." In this chapter I establish the groundwork of Judaism, concentrating on aspects of Jewish belief and practice that are relevant to both the cultural scene and my analysis. I also review American hat culture in order to further contextualize my study. In doing so, I form the foundation necessary for using Degel Israel as a starting point to consider more general patterns in Jewish congregational life. By examining the particular stresses and strains in the formation of identity in a small-town

Orthodox synagogue, I bring to the surface issues that affect a broad range of modern Jewish identities. This community is introduced in my third chapter, "Splitting Hairs: The Struggle for Community Definition in a Small Orthodox Synagogue." I investigate the difficulties of living in a small nonurban Orthodox community in a predominantly Christian area, including an exploration of the tensions that stem out of the lack of community definition. I argue that, although it is commonly assumed that rabbis are responsible for cultural and religious maintenance, it is the women of Degel Israel who ensure the survival of local Orthodox Jewry.

Small community Orthodox women exist on the periphery of their local community, Orthodoxy, and the academe. Their hair covering choices are especially individualized and are, at times, very surprising. This will be discussed at length in the fourth chapter, "Wearing Many Hats: The Hair Covering Practices of the Orthodox Jewish Women at Degel Israel Synagogue." I consider the women's self-identified motivations to cover their hair, as well as motivations that might exist outside of their awareness. My ultimate argument is that their applications of hair covering help to negotiate the tensions that they experience living in such a small religious community.

To present a contextualized consideration of hair covering, the following two chapters address nontraditional decisions made by Jewish women pertaining to their hair. In chapter five, "Letting Their Hair Down: Orthodox Women at Degel Israel Synagogue Who Choose Not to Cover Their Hair," I investigate the choices of some Orthodox women to forego hair covering. What I discover is that their hair covering choices are not as clearly defined as I had initially expected. For these women, there is a difference between observance and tradition. I argue that their behaviors and choices are regulated through an appreciation for and commitment to traditional Judaism. Chapter six, "Flipping Their Wigs for Judaism: Nonorthodox Women Who Choose to Cover Their Heads," represents a different point of view. These women do not have the same social pressures to cover their hair but take on a practice of covering their head, a decision that shapes their self-identity as a Jewish woman. I argue that although head covering is fundamentally different from hair covering, it still represents an empowering way that women communicate religious belief.

My work culminates with my conclusion in chapter seven, "The Long and Short of It: A Psychoreligious Interpretation of Hair Covering." In this chapter I discern patterns in the experiences of the various women profiled in my study and offer a psychoreligious interpretation of their covering practices. I synthesize the material gathered through ethnographic observation, interviews, and symbolic inventory and reveal the empowerment that their choice to cover (or not to cover) has instilled in them and consider what this means in light of their religious communities and concept of self. In addition, I probe the question of whether or not these women (and their choices) are responsible for the continuation of Orthodoxy and Judaism at large.

My analysis does not assume that Orthodox Jewish women are religiously oppressed. Rather, I probe questions of power and awareness of gender within Orthodox communities. I disagree with those who discount Orthodox women who cover their hair as being backwards or uneducated. Indeed, by choosing to cover their hair, these women have asserted a very external sign of their religious commitment. This demonstration of *Yiddishkeit* (Jewishness) drives my discussion of the powerful impact that hair covering can have for Jewish women. The continuum of hair covering can have a profound impact on those who choose to cover their hair. Covering practices become a marker of Jewish identity, the sisterhood which currently helps to define her, and how she will continue to be present for the future generations of women who come after her.

I give attention to hair as a separate subject in connection with Jewish culture by moving hair from the realms of religiously mandated dress to the forefront. I begin by exploring treatments of hair as a symbol, where consideration is given to psychoanalytic approaches to hair, as well as religious symbolism. The American and Jewish social systems are implicitly male-centered and assume a gendered binary of male/female.[4] My approach, however, does not dismiss factors of sexuality and gender identity. Following this psychoanalytic approach, I discuss hair as a marker, considering both secular and religious applications of hair marking. This is followed by a review of hair as an object, where I consider the importance of both male and female hair in Orthodox dress and garb. I conclude by using this foundation to assess the future potential for hair study and describe my methodology in hair theory.

HAIR AS SYMBOL

All of hair symbol study seems to lead back at some point to Charles Berg's publication, *The Unconscious Significance of Hair*.[5] Berg investigates the psychological importance that individuals unknowingly attribute to their hair. His work is heavily steeped in Freudian psychology, as he addresses the motivating factors that prompt hair styling and cutting. Relative to Freud, Berg considers human interaction with hair to represent universal repressed sexual thoughts. In other words, hair—both as a private and public symbol—represents one of the strongest links to sexuality in the human mind. Berg's analysis falls short, however, when one considers this argument for a universal psychoanalytic approach to hair. He fails to take into account both the social and cultural settings that affect hair customs. For example, while Berg argues that the phallic implications of hair have caused men to have short hair and women to have long hair, he does not consider other cultural norms which expect the opposite—for example, prior to Western influence, Native American men who were members of the Cherokee Nation grew their hair long, or Sikhs of both genders have long hair as a sign of their religious devotion.

Although Berg's assessment—that whenever an individual pays attention to hair, he or she expresses sexual pleasure—may be overstated and oversimplified, his work represents one of the first forays into hair scholarship and one of the few attempts to consider the psychological motivations for styling hair. The value in Berg's analysis rests not in his case studies—as they seem to be non-normative examples that he selected in order to support his point and are exclusively male—but in his general approach to hair as a profound link to the human subconscious. Although he does not consider any religious implications of hair, his theory can be easily applied to such investigations. Berg recognizes the link between hair and sexuality that, until his essay, was understood as either self-evident or nonimportant.

Berg's influence can clearly be seen in other works that consider the symbolism attached to hair. Anthropologist E. R. Leach's article, "Magical Hair" is a direct response to Berg's essay.[6] Leach considers hair to not only be demonstrative but also interactive; hair, in his view, represents both a public and a private symbol. Publicly, hair communicates identity and is, therefore, highly social. On the other hand, hair projects repressed anxieties and can both elicit emotion from individuals, as well as alter how they perceive themselves.

Leach concerns himself particularly with the presentation of an anthropological argument to contrast to Berg's psychoanalysis of hair. Although he affirms aspects of Berg's work—such as his understanding of hair as having the potential to serve as a phallic public symbol—Leach questions Berg's methods regarding cultural and social context. Berg ignores the nuances presented by Leach's more particular symbolic approach to hair, including the use of hair in head hunting, talismans, and relics. Leach's understanding of hair represents a more multifaceted and situated approach. He reminds readers that hair does not have one universal interpretation, and although he agrees that there are strong psychological ties between hair and sexuality, he places hair in a cultural continuum. This permits hair to function in a system of binaries. Rather than universalizing hair, a binary system allows hair to function as a dual symbol for wild/tame, public/private, social/individual, conservative/liberal, or unrestrained/restrained. As Leach suggests, universalizing hair is dangerous—psychology and culture must both be accounted for when considering the symbolic power of hair.

It is no surprise that Gananath Obeyesekere's anthropological work on Hindu hair symbolism relies heavily on Leach and Berg. His book, *Medusa's Hair: An Essay on Personal Symbols and Religious Experience,* is concerned primarily with the Hindu experience of matted locks.[7] Obeyesekere investigates Hindu ascetics, in particular women, who have cultivated long matted locks of hair that they understand to be imbued with religious sanctity. For these women, their matted hair was given to them by a deity and contains or embodies that deity's essence.

Obeyesekere applies Leach's methodology of placing hair in a situated context, as he sees these matted locks as personal symbols that have become public. That is to say, these symbols operate on an individual level pertaining to the wearer's relationship to a deity, but also are forced to function on a public level, as the wearer endures ridicule and pressure to remove the hair. He indicates that matted locks are only symbolically significant for the individual; outsiders assume a lack of personal hygiene and often chastise the wearer. However, beyond stemming from a deity's blessing, the matted locks come to symbolize for the individual an unwavering commitment to ascetic Hinduism.

Obeyesekere believes, in line with Leach, that these matted locks represent traditional symbols that are embedded both in religion and culture. Taken out of their cultural context, they are rendered ineffective and meaningless, which would seem to argue against Berg's universal psychoanalytic approach. Hindu culture, as Obeyesekere points out, is a shame-based culture in contrast with the Western Judeo-Christian guilt based cultures.[8] The binary of guilt and shame carries over into a comparison of individual and social symbols. In guilt based cultures, the emphasis is placed on the individual, thus rendering individualized symbol sets as particularly important. On the other hand, shame based cultures stress social perception, thereby necessitating greater navigation and understanding of public symbol sets. Based on this binary, individuals select symbol sets and maneuver within them to find forms of self-expression. Although Obeyesekere would agree that there is a profound psychological influence and impact when selecting and engaging with a symbol set and how it is used, he would disagree with Berg's approach of universalizing the utilized symbol sets. Matted locks, in this instance, function symbolically only when entrenched in Hindu culture.

Berg, Leach, and Obeyesekere taken together put forth an anthropological approach to hair as symbol. The importance of Berg's psychoanalytic approach should not be underestimated by his lack of attention to culture; however, it is important to understand Berg's argument in tandem with Leach's anthropological approach. The two present a holistic approach to hair symbolism that Obeyesekere employs in his consideration of Hindu matted locks. There is a danger inherent in both approaches—whether it is in assuming universal symbolism in the case of Berg or Leach's negation of the profound psychological influences of symbolism. It is only when the two approaches are combined that a method of hair symbolism emerges that takes into account both profound psychological motivations and the cultural setting and public understanding of hair. This methodology allows for hair to function dually as both a public and private symbol—yielding at times different results, as seen in Obeyesekere's work, for the implications of the private and public symbol.

HAIR AS MARKER

Theoretically, hair may also be understood as a significant marker of identity. We have just considered how hair can be symbolically viewed as functioning outside of the consciousness of the individual. In contrast, hair as a marker considers how individuals knowingly make choices about their hair and its appearance. In this approach, hair is utilized by the wearer as an indicator of status or of personal identity. It functions, essentially, as a form of self-expression. This understanding of hair is not rooted in deep symbolism or psychoanalysis. Rather, it yields hair as an ever changing marker of style, attitude, and personal choice.

Hair serves as a form of cultural expression, as well as personal style. Functioning as a marker, hair has several purposes. It is transformative, allowing individuals to mark change in themselves. It is performative when it functions as a showcase for public perception. Likewise, hair is situated, permitting others to identify individuals based on location, group allegiance, or events. Finally, hair functions as a behavioral marker, deeply entrenched in routine and daily maintenance. Taken together, this approach to hair concentrates more on the public marking of hair; it does, however, also allow for a deeply personal relationship to hair and hair styling.

Grant McCracken's book, *Big Hair: A Journey into the Transformation of Self*, claims that hair's significance lies in its transformative nature, serving as a form of self-invention.[9] His study concentrates on how women convey identity through hair. He notes that women make daily decisions to maintain certain hair styles, which he believes indicates to others how they wish to be perceived. Whether it is the cut, style, or color of hair, women make conscious choices as to the appearance of their hair; what these choices convey is embedded in their cultural setting and is highly public. Such a public statement is both temporary and performative. In other words, public displays of hair assume that coiffure will be seen by others that one is not familiar with; therefore, hair becomes a performative action through which the wearer is able to emphasize the individualized notion of self.

McCracken likens hair to the 1950s battle of the sexes, when uncontrolled hair mirrored feminine freedom, wildness, and expressiveness, and controlled hair represented compliance and restricted femininity.[10] As women began to experience sexual liberation, so did their hair. Perfectly coifed locks were previously associated with proper femininity; they gave way to unrestrained and flowing hair, which indicated a resistance to the patriarchal system. This serves as an example of how hair is easily changeable and very public, allowing women to engage in trends and use their hair to convey their beliefs or attitudes.

For McCracken, hair transcends fashion modes; it marks group identity. If a woman wishes to be perceived as sexy, chaste, professional, young, or high-class, she can alter her hair in an attempt to conform to the public perception of these groups. For example, a teenage girl who wishes to be perceived as different from her peers or misunderstood may use her hair as an external marker of her self-perceived angst by dying it black, growing it long, and having it hang over her eyes in a "goth" look. On the other hand, another teenager who wishes to be accepted into a more popular group of girls may dye her hair blonde and wear it in the same style that the high school cheerleaders are sporting. In both cases, these girls have made a conscious choice to use their hair as a public marker of how they envision themselves or wish to be perceived.

Although McCracken focuses more on how hair is publicly marked, Rose Weitz's book, *Rapunzel's Daughters: What Women's Hair Tells Us About Women's Lives*, illuminates the more personal side of hair marking.[11] Weitz agrees with McCracken's assessment, but she advances it by considering how hair emblematizes individuality. For example, when women feel that they are being controlled by patriarchy or by a particular male figure in their lives, they often still retain control over their hair and use it as a form of self-expression.[12] Likewise, hair can be used as a public marker of individual change. For example, when a woman chooses to shave her head upon entering a convent, she makes a conscious decision to alter her appearance in accordance with the substantial life change that she experiences.

Weitz explores the female attachment to hair beyond just color and style. She considers the empowerment that some Muslim women experience by choosing to privatize and cover their hair.[13] The veil, in this instance, becomes a public marker of religiosity and, at the same time, a private marker of personal spirituality and empowerment. Hair can also be used, as Weitz notes, as a marker of degradation. For example, when shaving the head of prisoners or mental patients, the individuals are stripped of their identity and deprived of their individuality; the hair that had served to mark them as unique has been taken away, and their individuality has been removed. The removal of hair can be seen as a punishment, as it was utilized, for example, during the Holocaust. Likewise, voluntary baldness is sometimes associated with aggression, as is the case with many professional boxers or soldiers.

Weitz does not, however, discuss the public marking of hair removal as a form of mourning. Although she admits that she is taking a decidedly American approach to hair study, she does, at times, weave in threads from other cultures. Her lack of mention of hair in the mourning processes seems a significant oversight. In line with her argument of hair removal as marking a fresh start, hair removal as part of mourning rituals also marks an external representation of status change; in this way individuals distinguish themselves as grieving and seek to externalize their internal anguish. [14]

Similar to Weitz's argument of hair marking the novitiate is Debra Renee Kaufman's analysis of hair and hair covering in *Rachel's Daughters: Newly Orthodox Jewish Women*. [15] As Kaufman considers women who have returned to or who have embraced Orthodoxy, she briefly considers their relationship with hair. Although Kaufman likely considers her approach to hair and hair covering as part of material culture, her treatment of hair renders it an expressive marker of religious devotion. She is not so much concerned with how, when, or by what means women cover their hair. Rather, she approaches hair as a demonstrable sign of Orthodox conversion to both the wearer and the viewer.

The women in Kaufman's case study use their hair as an entry point into Jewish ritual. As they move away from the secular world with which they are familiar, their hair marks them as decidedly Orthodox; it demonstrates an external commitment to leading an observant life. Many of the women interviewed state their distaste for what they perceive as a hypersexualized world. Through the reappropriation of their hair, which had previously represented their more worldly lifestyles, these women mark themselves as part of a religious community that is decidedly different from the hypersexualized culture they want to leave behind.

By covering their hair, these women accept a community marker of gendered difference. Many of them expressed to Kaufman their confusion over blurred gender roles in the secular world. For them, their hair helps negotiate and establish distinct gender roles. Their hair marks them as decidedly female and Orthodox to the outside community. Much of their engagement in Jewish ritual is private—for example, visiting the *mikveh* (ritual bath) or keeping a kosher home—but their hair marks them as a religious woman both to Orthodox community members as well as the secular world.

McCracken, Weitz, and Kaufman present a relatively full spectrum of hair marking. From McCracken's analysis of the blonde bombshell, to Weitz's treatment of shaving the head, and Kaufman's understanding of hair as a public marker of Jewishness, all three consider the profound impact that hair has on women. Their research lacks consideration of male hair. All three clearly state that they are investigating female topics—and in the case of Kaufman, hair factors only mildly in the grand scope of her project. However, one cannot help but wonder how their understanding of hair as a marker would have been enriched if they had extended their scope to include male appropriation of the same hair markers. For McCracken, his analysis of big hair would have been aided by the consideration of the popular male afro or of the mullet. Weitz ignores the public humiliation of the removal of *payot* (sidecurls) for Jewish men during the Holocaust. Although she includes men in her analysis of head shaving in the military, she ignores men when considering monasticism. Her argument about the novitiate would have been strengthened with consideration of regarding tonsuring and hair removal for monks. Similarly, Kaufman's discussion of changes in hair marking a lifestyle change for newly Orthodox women could also easily be applied to their male peers.

Many studies of the body ignore the importance of hair as a marker. However, as McCracken, Weitz, and Kaufman demonstrate, women utilize hair as an elaborate marker of how they wish to be perceived, as well as how they recognize themselves. Although Berg would likely point to this as a deeply embedded psychological desire to represent aspects of the subconscious, McCracken, Weitz, and Kaufman astutely portray hair as a malleable and ever changing cultural marker. Engaging in hair alteration is not always subconscious, as Berg suggests; rather, women change their hair to conform or to rebel against what is culturally expected. Through their use of hair as a marker of who they are or who they hope to be, women make a conscious choice to utilize their hair as an externalization of identity.

HAIR AS OBJECT

When scholars interpret hair, a third concept emerges that renders hair as one functional aspect in a range of material culture. In this view, hair becomes part of the uniform of a certain group and works in tandem with other costuming elements. This understanding is colored by both the group itself, as well as external perceptions of the group. Examples of this include ritualized hair styles of the military or religiously mandated hair styles as part of religious garb.

One example of this approach can be found in Solomon Poll's *The Hasidic Community of Williamsburg: A Study in the Sociology of Religion*.[16] Although he does not offer a comprehensive treatment of hair in his book, Poll considers hair as part of the general issue of community garb for Hasidim. He notes that all Hasidic men are marked as different through their distinctive modes of dress and through wearing *payot*; however, unmarried Hasidic women are not externally marked in the same way. It is not until they are married that their costume changes when they begin to cover their hair. He offers a hierarchy of Hasidic male dress that is based on religiosity and piety. For Poll, more traditional garb indicates a more conservative Hasidic worldview. He does not discuss varied applications of *payot*; rather, they seem to be an expected part of prescribed dress. Poll treats hair only in passing, as he focuses his understanding of Hasidic costuming on garments and neglects other elements of self-fashioning—namely hair, *payot*, and beards.

Barbara Goldman Carrell applies Poll's hierarchy of male dress to female head coverings in her article, "Hasidic Women's Head Coverings."[17] Her investigation centers upon the method by which Hasidic women cover their hair. Ranging from women who completely cover their hair with only a *tichel* (head scarf) to women who exclusively wear human hair *sheitels* (wigs), Carrell links the range of hair covering practices to religious piety. In her hierarchy, women who choose to entirely cover their hair in an obvious way—in this case, by using a *tichel*—represent the most religiously observant Hasidic women. On the other hand, women who desire to look more natural and cover with less obtrusive human hair wigs represent more liberal Hasidic women. She asserts, ". . . the different and ranked modes of Hasidic women's head coverings express, assert, or defend a woman's social position or level of cultural competence."[18] For Carrell, head coverings are an essential part of religious costuming and clearly represent group adherence.

Although Carrell aptly applies Poll's method, she ignores some of the cultural variations between Hasidic communities. It is generally true that, as Poll points out, that the more conservative the Hasidic court, the more conservative their garb; female head covering practices are heavily influenced by what is culturally acceptable within each Hasidic court. In other words, there is very little personal autonomy involved when a woman considers what her cultural group upholds as adequate hair covering. A more liberal woman may feel pressured by her religious in-laws to cover her hair by a different means when visiting them, but if she were to wear the same head covering among her own social circle, she might be chastised for appearing presumptuous. Carrell's argument would be well served if she took into consideration the influences of the Hasidic courts on mandated or expected garb. By ignoring this, she establishes a hierarchy without sound context. Likewise, her argument would be strengthened if she delved into other issues of modest dress as prescribed by individual Hasidic courts. By ignoring the link between head covering and *tznius* (modesty) practices—for example, the opaqueness of stockings—Carrell fails to situate her hair covering hierarchy in Hasidic material culture. Poll, on the other hand, grounds his hierarchy of male dress squarely in an understanding of variances of Hasidic courts and mandated dress patterns; however, he overlooks the importance of distinctive hair styling. If these two approaches could be joined, they would present a more encompassing overview of Hasidic garb and hair.

A well-rounded approach to Haredi religious garb is found in David Landau's *Piety and Power: The World of Jewish Fundamentalism.*[19] He tests the waters of cultural assimilation, noting that Hasidim historically made a conscious choice to appear different from the world around them, whereas other Orthodox Jews attempted to blend in. His analysis of this assimilation concentrates on the appropriation of *payot* by men, noting that Hasidim generally wear *payot* more prominently as a display of their religiosity.[20]

With their use of noticeable *payot*, these men render their hair as part of the expected costuming of their group. While arguments can be made for *payot* as both religious markers and public/private symbols, in Landau's work they represent a religious item—much like *tzitzit* (fringes worn by observant men)—that are created and upheld by individuals as part of their faith.

Landau also analyzes changes in religious dress as a step made by those who join ultraorthodox groups. Through their change in dress, these new members assert their belonging. Although this could also be seen as a marker, as it is in the case of Kaufman, Landau approaches changes in hair and dress as part of accepting an expected pattern of dress and group identification. In this case, *payot* are created or cultivated and maintained.

Orthodox women also utilize *sheitels* as a form of observant dress. At present, the most expansive treatment of *sheitel* use can be found in Pesach Eliyahu Falk's *Sheitels: A Halachic Guide to Present-Day Sheitel.*[21] Falk, an expert on Jewish law, offers a critique of how Orthodox women engage with their hair coverings. Unlike his other works in which he concentrates on interpretation and implementation of rabbinic law, here he is interested in not when or why women cover, but how. He admonishes readers to, "SOS!"—Save Our *Sheitels*![22] Falk expects a general understanding from readers that hair covering is essential and is a logical outgrowth of *tznius*; his concern is that women are choosing to wear immodest *sheitels* in an attempt to appear more natural.

Falk blends religious law with material culture. It is not enough for a woman to simply cover her hair; if she appears to be uncovered, she still risks sexually enticing men. In this way, Falk creates a binary gendered relationship to Jewish garb. In his understanding, Orthodox men wear their costume and hair as a uniform, but pious women wear a dress of distinction. In other words, Orthodox men's dress demonstrates their affiliation. Women's dress, on the other hand, is spiritual and becomes part of their perceived holiness. Their clothes are more expressive and less uniform, and because of this, it is possible for women to play more with the boundaries of modesty. Falk's treatment of *sheitels* attempts to codify a set of rules and regulations for women, as well as serve as a warning of the dangers of appearing too secular. Dress and hair, in the case of Falk, prove themselves as regulators of group cohesion.[23]

Approaching hair as an object of material culture is helpful in fostering an understanding of its role in religious garb and costuming, but danger also lurks beneath the surface. Material culture approaches to hair ignore the profound emotional attachment that individuals have to their hair. Likewise, hair is an outgrowth of the body, and while it may be shaped or removed, it regenerates; hair texture, growth patterns, and color are predetermined in a way that most material culture items are not. Hair is organic and not a human construction. This makes it difficult to negotiate for many scholars interested in material culture, which perhaps helps to explain why hair has been so overlooked. Certainly consideration of hair as part of mandated or created costuming is important, but its implications should not be limited by the constraints of this methodology. That is to say, material culture studies should include the interpretation of hair, but scholars of hair should branch out of material culture and also include other investigations of the more emotional aspects of hair.

THE FUTURE OF HAIR STUDY: A HYBRID METHODOLOGY

Although the works reviewed in this chapter demonstrate an understanding of the importance of hair for individuals, the impact that hair has had within religious groups still remains under-surveyed and under-theorized. It seems, at best, that hair finds itself encapsulated in passing remarks about religious material culture, or in psychoanalytic approaches of hair as symbol, as is the case with Obeyesekere's work. Hair has been overlooked because it is too familiar, making it difficult for scholars to externalize or objectify for analysis. Hair study is subsumed under either costume or bodylore, failing to take into account that while hair functions in both of these areas, it also warrants separate attention for cultural formation.

My own investigation of hair focuses on women and Jews as subjects in comparison and contrast to general American Christian society, taking into consideration worldviews suggested by both outsiders and Jews. Despite this narrow scope, my entry point into hair study begins in a more general way with an effort to make the familiar strange. Hair has become such an accepted part of contemporary bodylore that it has been glossed over. By spotlighting the cultural role of hair, I hope that something that is so familiar can be reevaluated for the deep and rich symbolism it expresses.

The lack of a comprehensive study of hair covering suggests a general misconception that either significant investigations of Jewish hair already exist or that hair is unimportant in religious dialogue. Likewise, virtually no literature exists pertaining to nonorthodox women who choose to cover their hair or heads. There are two ways that this manifests itself—through full hair covering as seen in Orthodox circles but applied in a nonorthodox setting and women who choose to wear *kippot* when taking part in religious services or events. In both instances I see a strong association with the ritualization of hair or head covering and the act of religious or social female empowerment.

As I study hair, I blend the three above methods, creating a hybrid methodology that allows for hair to function as a religious symbol, a religious marker, and as an object in religious material culture. In particular, I am interested in how hair is utilized to create, maintain, and blend boundaries, both within and outside of the Orthodox community. Such a study is attuned not only to socially constructed religious boundaries, but also includes gender, secular, familial, and social boundaries. Hair as a religious marker represents a clear application of both symbolic and material culture aspects of hair within Orthodoxy. The intentionality of hair as a symbol and marker is not quite as clear. Do women intentionally use their hair or is it subconscious? Are women working within an inherited material culture system or symbolic set, or are they deliberately conceptualizing their hair?

Americans freely throw around terms like Freudian, psychoanalyze, and neurotic. As these terms enter popular discourse, their application to real life is often lost. For the purposes of this investigation, I apply the neo-Freudian concepts of Erich Fromm to my study because of his greater attention to religion, which makes his framework more applicable to my study than Freud, Horney, Bettelheim, or Erikson. He identifies psychoanalysis as the understanding that our behavior, thoughts, and desires are governed by processes outside of our awareness, generally considered subconscious. Therefore, when we try to consciously evaluate these processes, we resist or struggle to bring them into our consciousness. Some psychoanalysts, like Sigmund Freud and Carl Jung, believe that thought and behavioral development are set in childhood. Likewise, when our view of reality conflicts with our subconscious desires or needs, we are prone to experience neurotic effects (depression, anxiety, obsession). To negotiate these tensions, psychoanalysis seeks to bring the subconscious and conscious into harmony.[24] For this study, I am not concerned with the clinical use of psychoanalysis but its application to social and cultural situations.[25]

Within psychoanalysis, there are many different branches or approaches to its application—including, but not limited to, object relations theory, self-psychology, cultural psychoanalysis, relational psychoanalysis, and interpersonal psychoanalysis. The psychoanalytical approach used in my analysis is in line with cultural psychoanalysis. This approach allows for culture, particularly the culture in which one is raised, to factor into the formation of the mind and human behavior.[26] The importance of this cultural revision is the idea that mental processes are not universal but situated in cultural contexts. Alan Dundes argues that Freud, despite being credited with suggesting that symbols, customs, and folklore arise out of the projection of anxieties, assumed a basis of psychic unity that does not account for cultural context.[27]

Cultural psychoanalysis is generally considered neo-Freudian. Neo-Freudians are influenced by the work of Freud, using the core ideas of projection, subconscious (especially the important sociological notion of the superego), stages of development, and primacy of gender, but ply a more socially and culturally contextualized approach to adult (as opposed to Freud's concentration on childhood) normal conduct in everyday life. Included in this neo-Freudian approach is questioning universalistic, masculinist concepts such as penis envy and a move toward being attuned to culture.[28] As Erich Fromm explains, traditional psychoanalysts "did not concern themselves with the variety of life experience . . . and therefore did not try to explain psychic structure as determined by social structure."[29] For cultural psychoanalysts, society and culture cannot and should not be separated from the self. Rather, when considering the conscious and subconscious, analysts should include consideration of the embedded cultural assumptions, beliefs, and practices of the individual.

In using cultural psychoanalysis in this study, I am aware of the critique of the superego effect the determinative factor of society writ small. Levels of cultural influence can be sorted into small group, community, or nationality. If all of these factors are at work, how are they manifested differently or simultaneously through performance? In my study, I question the significance of the congregation as a social structure for the development of a cultural personality in relation to others, including Lancaster as a small city, America as a nation-state, and Judaism as a religious community. I believe that cultural psychoanalysis has concentrated on the white, Western, heterosexual, male experienced because that has traditionally been the life-experience of those trained in psychoanalysis.[30] Traditional psychoanalysts have felt most qualified or interested in reflecting on their own life experiences, considering other cultures or social motivations "nonnormative." By stepping outside of this paradigm, I suggest that when approaching less familiar cultural groups, it is crucial to acknowledge that what may seem strange to individuals in one culture is normative for another.

Hair has become increasingly important for religious women. Although there exists a long history of female head covering within Judaism, it is only in the last two or three generations of Jewish women that the issue has become a topic of discussion. The reasons for this are likely multifaceted. Previous generations of Jewish women lived in relative (or literal) ghettoization. They lead isolated lives that were defined by otherness. As Judaism evolved into a more urban religion (approximately after 1880), and as these women left their isolated small communities, the pressure to conform and assimilate increased. As previously mentioned, while Orthodox male dress is uniform in nature, women experienced greater flexibility with their clothing choices. As their garments became more assimilated, it is no wonder that their hair followed suit.

As Judaism continued to develop in urban areas, it underwent additional cultural changes. It no longer was economically practical for men to study all day and for wives to remain at home. Women entered the work force (approximately after 1950), often finding employment with secular businesses. As these women ventured out of Orthodox enclaves, they were bombarded with images of the contemporary American woman. Once again, assimilation influenced their head-covering choices. Likewise, with the demise of

American hat culture, the pressures to bareheaded increased as a response to new American cultural norms.[31]

When considering Degel Israel, which is admittedly a small community sample, it is critical to evaluate how lessons learned can be transferred to larger studies. Degel Israel's small size does not equate to small issues. Rather, they are confronted with the same difficulties and questions as contemporary American Jews. However, instead of having the option of splintering into subgroups, they must face these difficulties head on and negotiate them as a community. There are numerous examples of this—including the celebration of bat mitzvahs, as discussed in chapter three, or the acceptance of a variety of levels of religious observance.

Congregational studies have generally taken two approaches: demographic or historical. There is value in each approach, but neither investigates the process of a congregation. Demographics and statistics tell us what is happening but do not ask why. Historical approaches tell us what happened, but fail to ask how congregants perceived its happening. Through my ethnographic approach, in addition to considering history and demographics, I am attuned to the congregational process with questions such as how did this happen and how did you make it happen? Congregational studies have traditionally assumed a tendency toward secularization; however, they fail to explain contemporary renewed interest in Orthodox Judaism or the ways in which communities have defied secularization. Because the membership of Degel Israel offers a limited sample size, I have drawn in other congregational studies to offer comparison. Building on this foundation, my extensive interviews of the women of Degel Israel provide depth and perspective. In this study, I attempt to draw out the negotiations and practices that result from the necessary tensions caused by holding a small congregation together. What emerges is the voice of struggling Jewish synagogues across America. They share commonalities like decreased membership, financial hardship, geographic isolation, low retention rates, and aging members. Although their geographic situation in Amish country is unique, Degel Israel's struggle to define itself and negotiate traditionalism with assimilation is representative of the American Orthodox experience.

Historic and demographic studies have approached small town Jewry in three ways: they have blurred small town and suburbia, they have assumed progressive rather than traditional affiliation within small communities, or they have predicted the ultimate demise of small town synagogues.

One common approach to nonurban Jews is to consider them suburban. However, as demonstrated in studies such as Albert Gordon's *Jews in Suburbia,* Etan Diamond's *And I Will Dwell in their Midst: Orthodox Jews in Suburbia,* and Marshall Sklare's *Jewish Identity on the Suburban Frontier*, suburban experiences do not equate to small town life.[32] Although there certainly are lifestyle differences—warranting studies of suburban Jews separately from urban Jews—suburban Jews are still afforded access to Jewish culture and connections in the general metropolitan area. Urban Jews live in greater concentration and do not experience the same isolation as Jews in small communities. They can choose between synagogues, have Jewish colleagues, and can expect that their children will meet other Jewish children at school. From the small town Jewish vantage point, suburban Jews are essentially urban.

Other studies, such as Gerald Lee Showstack's *Suburban Communities: The Jewishness of American Reform Jews,* assume that small town Jewish communities are progressive and decidedly unorthodox. [33] Others, like Peter Rose's *Strangers in Their Midst: Small-Town Jews and Their Neighbors,* include passages to substantiate this claim, such as, "I was raised in an Orthodox home. When we first came here we kept kosher, but after a while we gave that up. . . . We still belong to a synagogue where I grew up, but we only attend on the high holidays." [34] Chapter three will address the tendency for small communities to affiliate with the Reform movement, but the experiences of small town Orthodoxy should not be ignored because they buck the trend of progressivism.

Finally, studies of small town Jews have generally assumed their eventual demise. Rose writes in 1958, that "the small-town Jew is in reality a disappearing type in the spectrum of American Jewry." [35] He reevaluates this in the 1977 edition of his book, saying, "In time to come it will be hard to find isolated Jews in rural Gentile communities, Jews who are, *de facto,* strangers in their midst." [36] Similarly, Lee Levinger writes in 1952, "Thus, as time passes, it seems that we shall soon have to write off most of the 150,000 village Jews from the roster of American Jewry." [37] Yet, over half a century later, nearly 15 percent of American Jewry is living in small communities. [38] It may not be easy and trends may still point to their decline, but clearly they are negotiating the tensions of their minority status and are surviving outside of urban areas. [39]

In evaluating this survival, it is critical to listen to the women's voices. Their experiences are rife with the tension between traditionalism and assimilation. Congregational studies, like the work done by Jack Kugelmass in *The Miracle of Intervale Avenue: The Story of a Jewish Congregation in the South Bronx,* have generally focused on the male experience, assuming maleness as normative for synagogue life. [40] This undergirds the traditional idea of Jewish women's responsibility for Judaism in the home and Jewish men's role of public observance. However, as I demonstrate, albeit submerged at times, it is the women's roles at home and in congregational life that allow Orthodoxy to survive.

My ethnographic approach to Orthodox hair covering begins by investigating the hair covering practices of the women of Degel Israel Synagogue, a small nonurban community of Orthodox Jews in Lancaster, Pennsylvania. By bringing a psychoanalytical approach together with cultural and societal perceptions, and merging it with a congregational analysis through a gendered lens, I probe the transformative power of hair. I combine this understanding with the religious resources available and the words and opinions of local Orthodox women, constructing an argument based on a psychoreligious analysis of the impact that hair has within religious communities and for individuals. By taking into account the basic hierarchy model established by Poll and Carrell and expanding it to include a variety of hair and head covering practices, I also attempt to negotiate the impact of cultural and societal influences on hair covering. In doing so, I engage hair covering in a more encompassing way that takes into consideration *minhag*, religious tradition, and changes in American cultural norms. By making hair central to my inquiry, I hypothesize that hair covering represents an external sign of personal dedication to Judaism that manifests the empowerment Jewish women, particularly those in small communities, often unknowingly experience through their engagement with hair covering—an empowerment that is crucial for the survival of small town Orthodoxy.

NOTES

1. America's Next Top Model. Season 14, episode 2. First broadcast March 17, 2010 by The CW Network. Produced by Tyra Banks, Ken Mok, and Daniel Soiseth.

2. In particular, Islamic head covering has received increased attention due to recent political questions of the separation of church and state. Muslim women worldwide have been faced with legal ramifications as governments have legislated that they are only allowed to cover their heads in certain ways. Within the United States, Islamic veiling has come into question in terms of company uniforms, sports team uniforms, and professional dress code.

3. A word about transliteration—all Hebrew words have been transliterated according to the common Sephardic transliteration style. However, the women interviewed frequently used Yiddish or Ashkenazic pronunciation—for example, the substitution of a "t" with an "s," as in *tallit/tallis*. When transliterating Yiddish, I have followed the common Ashkenazic pronunciation. However, when quoting from printed sources, I have left the author's original spelling unaltered. Certain words have been italicized and, in addition to in-text glosses, are also included in a glossary appendix to help the reader.

4. See Mari Jo Buhle, *Feminism and Its Discontents: A Century of Struggle with Psychoanalysis* (Cambridge, MA: Harvard University Press, 2000); Juliet Mitchell and Sangay Mishra, *Psychoanalysis and Feminism: A Radical Reassessment of Freudian Psychoanalysis* (New York: Basic Books, 1974); Nancy Chodorow, *Feminism and Psychoanalytic Theory* (New Haven: Yale University Press, 1991).

5. Charles Berg, *The Unconscious Significance of Hair* (London: George Allen and Unwin, 1951).

6. E. R. Leach, "Magical Hair," *The Journal of the Royal Anthropological Institute of Great Britain and Ireland* 88 (July–December 1958): 147–64.

7. Gananath Obeyesekere, *Medusa's Hair: An Essay on Personal Symbols and Religious Experience* (Chicago: University of Chicago Press, 1984).

8. Obeyesekere, *Medusa's Hair*, 80-81.

9. Grant McCracken, *Big Hair: A Journey into the Transformation of Self* (Woodstock, NY: Overlook Press, 1995).

10. McCracken, *Big Hair*, 36.

11. Rose Weitz, *Rapunzel's Daughters: What Women's Hair tells Us About Women's Lives* (New York: Farrar, Straus and Giroux, 2004).

12. Weitz, *Rapunzel's Daughters*, 104.

13. Weitz, *Rapunzel's Daughters*, 110.

14. Marcia Pointon, "Materializing Mourning: Hair, Jewellery, and the Body, in *Fashion: Critical and Primary Sources: The Nineteenth Century*, ed. Peter McNeil (Oxford, UK: Berg, 2009), 345–58.

15. Renee Kaufman, *Rachel's Daughters: Newly Orthodox Jewish Women* (New Brunswick, NJ: Rutgers University Press, 1991).

16. Solomon Poll, *The Hasidic Community of Williamsburg: A Study in the Sociology of Religion* (New York: Free Press, 1962).

17. Barbara Goldman Carrell, "Hasidic Women's Head Coverings" in *Religion, Dress, and the Body*, ed. Linda B. Arthur (Oxford, UK: Oxford University Press, 1999), 163–80.

18. Carrell, "Hasidic Women," 174.

19. David Landau, *Piety and Power: The World of Jewish Fundamentalism* (New York: Hill and Wang, 1992).

20. Landau, *Piety and Power*, 19–34.

21. Pesach Eliyahu Falk, *Sheitels: A Halachic Guide to Present-Day Sheitels* (Jerusalem: Bnos Melochim, 2002).

22. Falk, *Sheitels*, 15.

23. See Margaret Reynolds, *Plain Women: Gender and Ritual in the Old Order River Brethren* (University Park: Pennsylvania State University Press, 2001).

24. Erich Fromm, *Die Entdeckung des gesellschaftlichen Unbewussten: Zur Neubestimmung der Psychoanalyse* (Weinheim, Germany: Beltz, 1990), 12–16.

25. This is in line with the work of Anna Freud, who helped move psychoanalysis toward the study of the normal in everyday life.

26. José Guimón, *Relational Mental Health: Beyond Evidence-Based Interventions* (New York: Springer, 2004), 59–82.

27. Alan Dundes, *Parsing Through Customs: Essays by a Freudian Folklorist* (Madison: University of Wisconsin Press, 1987).

28. Hellmuth Benesch, "Neu-Psychoanalyse," in *Enzyklopädisches Wörterbuch Klinische Psychologie und Psychotherapie*, ed. Hellmuth Benesch (Weinheim, Germany: Beltz, 1995), 550–70.

29. Adam Philips, *On Flirtation* (Cambridge, MA: Harvard University Press, 1996), 132.

30. See Gilles Deleuze and Felix Guattari, *Anti-Oedipus: Capitalism and Schizophrenia* (Minneapolis: University of Minnesota Press, 1983), 159–62.

31. See Hasia Diner, *The Jews of the United States: 1654–2000* (Berkeley: University of California Press, 2006); Colin McDowell, *Hats: Status, Style, and Glamour* (New York: Rizzoli, 1992); Neil Steinberg, *Hatless Jack: The President, the Fedora, and the History of American Style* (New York: Plume, 2004).

32. Albert Gordon, *Jews in Suburbia* (Boston: Beacon Press, 1959); Etan Diamond, *And I Will Dwell in their Midst: Orthodox Jews in Suburbia* (Chapel Hill: University of North Carolina Press, 2000); Marshall Sklare, *Jewish Identity on the Suburban Frontier: A Study of Group Survival in the Open Society* (Chicago: University of Chicago Press, 1967).

33. Gerald Lee Showstack, *Suburban Communities: The Jewishness of American Reform Jews* (New York: Scholars Press, 1988).

34. Peter Rose, *Strangers in Their Midst: Small-Town Jews and Their Neighbors* (New York: Richwood Publishing, 1977).

35. Rose, *Strangers in Their Midst*, 158.

36. Rose, *Strangers in Their Midst*, 159.

37. Lee J. Levinger, "The Disappearing Small-Town Jew," *Commentary* 14 (July–December, 1952): 1961–62.

38. United Jewish Communities, "Jews in Small Communities," 2011, http://www.jewishfederations.org/local_includes/downloads/5542.pdf (accessed June 23, 2011), 3.

39. See Robert S. Lynd and Helen Merrell Lynd, *Middletown: A Study in Modern American Culture* (New York, Harcourt Brace Javanovich, 1959).

40. Jack Kugelmass, *The Miracle of Intervale Avenue: The Story of a Jewish Congregation in the South Bronx* (New York: Columbia University Press, 1996).

Chapter Two

Covering Jewish Women

The Congregational Context

Friends and colleagues are often surprised to learn that I spent two years studying Judaism in Marburg, Germany. Beyond scriptural and linguistic study, which I did alongside of other traditional theology students, a great deal of my time was spent studying with a retired rabbi. He offered one class each semester on Jewish topics, in which I always took part. Beyond that, we studied privately together. We joked about being an unlikely *chavrusa* (learning pair), but the reality was that I was his student—although he did enjoy practicing his English skills with me from time to time.

As I began exploring Orthodoxy in a small community, he shared with me that observant German Jews assume that all American Orthodox Jews live in urban communities that offer support and opportunities. He was skeptical that small community Orthodoxy was truly unurban. Our conversations have progressed along with my research, and the lifestyles of observant German Jews are remarkably similar to the experiences of small community American Jews. Separated from other observant Jews and living in Christian contexts, these groups are forced to constantly grapple with secularization, the feeling of otherness, and the difficult logistics of living observantly. Although I did not realize it at the time, my years spent studying in Marburg, Germany, profoundly influenced how I listened to the voices of American Jews. Those years taught me to seek out the stories of the marginalized, to look beyond urban centers, and to recognize that urban American Judaism does not define the entire American Jewish experience.

In this chapter I work toward establishing the foundation necessary to contextualize my ethnographic study of the women at Degel Israel Synagogue. I begin by introducing the four main movements of American Juda-

ism. For those familiar with Judaism, this will be review. However, understanding certain central tenets of Judaism establishes the foundation for readers that will be relevant throughout my study as I discuss the practices and
beliefs expressed by the women of Degel Israel. Following this, I explain the
practice of Jewish hair covering as well as American hat culture. Taken
together, these elements establish the necessary American historical, religious, and the cultural texts I observed in my study.

THE FOUR PILLARS OF FAITH AND THE MAJOR AMERICAN JEWISH MOVEMENTS

Jews are an ethnoreligious group, meaning that one can be a Jew by virtue of
ancestry or through spiritual belief. Typically, Jewish identity is a combination of both ethnic or cultural affiliation and religious belief. In order to best
understand the women profiled in this study, it is important to identify the
four pillars of Judaism—covenant, Torah, Sabbath, and *kashrut*—as well as
the four main movements of American Judaism: Orthodox, Conservative,
Reconstructionist, and Reform.[1]

Judaism is a covenantal religion. Jews believe that they are in a covenantal relationship with God and that as the "children of Israel," they are in fact
the "chosen people."[2] As the first monotheistic religion in the Ancient Near
East, Jews believe that when God was revealed to Moses on Sinai,[3] as well as
other instances throughout the Hebrew Bible,[4] God demonstrated that Jews
were chosen as God's special nation. This feeling of covenant has proven
invaluable in light of the Jewish Diaspora. Regardless of where Jews were
exiled and despite living scattered across the world, Jewish communities
retained the mindset that there still was one concrete Jewish covenantal body.
That is to say, despite secondary cultural identifications, it was their covenantal relationship with Judaism and God that has helped Jews maintain their
religious and cultural affiliation with Judaism.

This covenantal relationship is described throughout Jewish scripture but
is perhaps the most prominent in the Torah.[5] In this context, the Torah, also
known as the Pentateuch by biblical scholars, comprises the first Five Books
of Moses: Genesis, Exodus, Leviticus, Numbers, and Deuteronomy. The
Torah functions as the foundational Jewish text and religious document.
Central to Jewish belief is the idea that God communicated not only the
covenant but also God's expectations and commandments through the Torah.
Including the familiar Ten Commandments, the Torah has a total of 613
commandments that describe the various laws which Jews must follow. From
circumcision, forbidden foods, and ritualized behavior to the command for
charity and rest on the Sabbath, the crux of Jewish belief is following the

Torah and how literally to adhere to it as a guide of values or a body of directives.[6]

In addition to the *mitzvot* (commandments) found in the Torah, Jews uphold other religious laws, referred to as *halakha* (Jewish law). *Halakhic* regulations govern not only religious practice but also daily life. Jewish law not only stems from the Torah but also includes long-standing customs, as well as rabbinic laws and commentary. Taken together, *halakha* is an organic body of rules that is open to interpretation and has changed with time. Often Jews turn to rabbinic authorities for help interpreting *halakha*. However, the application and interpretation of *halakha* can vary by region, group identity, and individual preference.

Beyond being scripture and containing the *mitzvot*, the Torah also has a ritual function. On Saturday mornings during the Jewish Sabbath, a section of the Torah is read out loud. This is done consecutively through the year, including readings done on certain holidays. During the course of the Jewish calendar year, the entire Torah is read aloud.

The Torah reading is a crucial part of the Sabbath service, just as the Sabbath is an integral part of Jewish life. The Sabbath (also called *Shabbat*, from the Hebrew, and *Shabbos*, from the Yiddish) is observed from sunset on Friday evening until three stars can be seen in the sky on Saturday night. Jews celebrate the Sabbath as a day of rest that is mandated by God.[7] During *Shabbat*, time is spent with family, in the synagogue, resting, and studying scripture. Contemporary *Shabbat* observance varies from those who are *shomer shabbos* (strictly observant of the Sabbath)—who refuse to drive, carry items, write, or engage in any other type of work—to those who attend services but do not vary their weekend plans or lifestyle. Jewish liturgy describes the Sabbath as a taste of *olam haba* (the time after the Messiah) that also commemorates the Israelites redemption from Egyptian slavery. The Sabbath is a time to reflect and refocus on one's relationship with God. For many contemporary Jews, the Sabbath is a time to reconnect with their family, recharge themselves, and spend time reconnecting with God and/or their local Jewish community.[8]

Finally, Orthodox Jews place emphasis on *kashrut*. These are the set of Jewish dietary laws that are in accordance with *halakha*. Many of these laws come from Leviticus and Deuteronomy, although they have been expanded upon and interpreted throughout rabbinic texts. Within kosher cookery, there are three categories of kosher food: meat (Yiddish, *fleischig*; Hebrew, *basari*), dairy (Yiddish, *milchig*; Hebrew, *halavi*), and *parve* (Yiddish, *parev*, meaning neutral; the category includes fish, fruits, vegetables, and spices). Keeping a kosher kitchen and eating only kosher food is no easy task. It includes avoiding forbidden meats (including rabbit, pig, shellfish, and birds of prey), only eating meats that have been slaughtered according to kosher laws, separating meat and dairy (not only in consumption but also including the separation of utensils, cookware, flatware, dishes, and food storage containers), and avoiding foods that are not certified kosher (including not only foods in grocery stores but also restaurants).[9] Even more liberal Jews who do not keep kosher kitchens often stay away from certain foods—most commonly pig products and shellfish.

For Jews who keep strictly kosher, particularly for those who live in areas with few Jews, food preparation and consumption are constant concerns. Not only is it difficult to locate and purchase appropriate foodstuffs, but maintaining a kosher home is difficult in terms of floor plan and layout. Many observant Jews prefer having a kitchen with two separate sinks, two dishwashers, and increased cabinet space to house duplicate utensils, plates, pots and pans, and food storage containers. In areas like Lancaster, Pennsylvania, where homes are not built to accommodate kosher kitchens, there is considerable expense to physically alter layouts of home and kitchen.

Similarly, when choosing a home, observant Jews are also attuned to location and space. They must live in a home that is within walking distance to the local Orthodox synagogue. In small communities, this can pose significant problems. Whether it is an undesirable part of the city or the lack of adequate housing, location can be extremely limiting. To erect a *Sukkah* (a walled structure covered with branches) in which to eat, celebrate, and entertain guests during the Jewish holiday Sukkot, it is necessary to have enough space around the perimeter of one's home, or in line with many urban Jews, a porch on which to erect a Sukkah. As a result, observant Jews must not only struggle to find homes in an adequate location, but they also find themselves needing to alter their homes to accommodate the physical demands of both holidays and *kashrut*.

These variations in observance factor heavily into why American Judaism has broken into four major movements: Orthodox, Conservative, Reconstructionist, and Reform. All of the movements affirm several key points: monotheism, *klal Yisrael* (the responsibility for the Jewish community), and reliance on Jewish scripture. Where they diverge, however, is in levels of observance and egalitarianism.

Historically there were no branches of Judaism. Rather, Judaism itself was a singular affiliation. Outside of North America and Israel, this is still often the case. In Germany, for example, there are a variety of levels of Jewish observance. However, there are so few Jews that they typically do not identify with separate strains of Judaism. American Judaism, however, has evolved into several different movements, and even within those movements there are distinctions.[10]

Orthodox Judaism is the most traditional branch of Judaism. The movement itself is not overseen by any one particular rabbinic body, meaning that Orthodoxy is largely dependent on congregational leadership.[11] Orthodox Jews are the most observant of Jews and believe that the Torah and the Oral

Laws were given directly from God to Moses. These laws are the central tenets of their lives and govern most of their actions. For example, most Orthodox Jews keep strictly kosher, wear head/hair coverings, and uphold Sabbath laws. [12]

Within Orthodoxy there are several subgroups. The differentiation between these groups is key to understanding how Degel Israel Synagogue functions. The three primary subcategories are Modern Orthodoxy, Haredi Judaism, and Hasidic Judaism. [13] Modern Orthodoxy, which will be discussed at length in chapter five, upholds traditional Jewish law without completely removing oneself from the secular world. Modern Orthodox Jews tend to look more assimilated in terms of dress. Likewise, they engage freely with the secular world insofar as their religious obligations will allow. [14] On the other hand, Haredi Jews, also called ultraorthodox, advocate less secular involvement. They seek minimal engagement with contemporary society and tend to appear more separate in their dress. [15] Hasidic Jews, who could also be considered ultraorthodox, are similar in their desire to remove themselves from the secular world. However, they differ in their emphasis on Jewish mysticism. They, too, appear unassimilated in terms of dress and, when in the synagogue, engage in much more emotional prayer. [16]

Conservative Judaism, sometimes also called Masorti Judaism, took hold in the United States in the early 1900s. After Reform Judaism, which originated in Germany, split from Orthodoxy, Conservative Judaism represented the middle ground for Jews who wanted to both embrace more liberal practice but still retain tradition. Conservative Jews today are divided between egalitarian and non-egalitarian synagogues. Both rely more heavily on Hebrew in liturgy than Reform congregations, and congregants are more likely to uphold ritual observance, including the donning of *tallisim* (prayer shawls) and *kippot*. [17]

Reconstructionist Judaism broke off from Conservative Judaism in the 1980s. This is the smallest of the Jewish movements and is based on the teachings of Mordecai Kaplan (1881–1983). Reconstructionist Jews do not consider *halakha* binding, but rather something that needs to be updated and modernized. This approach allows for Jewish rituals and customs to significantly evolve, while still valuing the traditions typically associated with Judaism. Reconstructionist Jews believe that individuals should seek to incorporate Judaism into all aspects of their lives unless there is good reason not to do so. In this view, the *mitzvot* (commandments) are considered with rituals or folkways. This mindset allows for the maintenance of some tradition (Hebrew liturgy, wearing *kippot* and *tallisim*, studying of Torah) without a sense of binding obligation for those who do not find the practices spiritually enriching. [18]

Finally, Reform Judaism, sometimes also called Progressive Judaism, is a movement that began in Germany but gained prominence in the United

States. Reform Jews believe that Judaism should be thoroughly modernized and completely compatible with its surrounding culture. Reform Jews are, in many ways, the least ritually observant. However, that is not to negate their participation in Jewish life. The movement places a large emphasis on social justice and is very progressive in its stance on homosexuality, intermarriage, and patrilineal descent. Most Reform Jews have abandoned the practice of *kashrut* and many forego *kippot* and *tallisim.*[19]

THE SIGNIFICANCE OF JEWISH HAIR COVERING

Within Western religious traditions, uncut female hair has traditionally represented a conflicting symbol of both virginity and sexuality. This dichotomy manifests in Judaism as female hair covering after marriage. In choosing to cover, these women uphold tradition and embrace their new status of Jewish wife, and eventually, Jewish mother. Although this tradition is regarded as old fashioned and "old world" by most contemporary Western Jews, it is still practiced by Orthodox women. It continues to set these women apart as members of a subculture existing within the larger context of both American culture and American Judaism.

Although those not steeped in Orthodox Judaism frequently assume that hair covering stems from a biblical mandate, the Bible is surprisingly silent on this issue.[20] Hair covering for Jewish women stems from *minhag* (from the Biblical Hebrew, literally for "driving" [2 Kings 9:20]; understood in modern Jewish tradition as a custom representing a cultural norm) and is prescribed in subsequent rabbinic literature. Publications on *minhag* in Jewish tradition serve as more than just general religious commentary. Through a codification of culture, they have become the guidelines and rules for living an observant life, which has been particularly important for the diasporic culture of Judaism. In the case of hair covering, its mention in these rabbinic texts renders it essential for Orthodox women.

Historical precedence for hair covering develops perhaps as early as Ancient Near Eastern times (3100–330 BCE), as women in ancient Israel, as well as those living in the later Roman era, traditionally veiled themselves when in public spaces.[21] This represents, however, the standard for all women of the time and not those associated with a particular religion, making it difficult to discern whether traditional hair covering was understood to be part of local culture or if Jews at the time also understood it as religious obligation. During the Middle Ages most women continued to cover their hair.[22] However, Medieval Jews in Germanic lands stood apart from their contemporaries, as they were forced to wear a *Judenhut*—a yellow cone-like hat that distinguished Jews when outside of the sanctioned ghetto. The *Judenhut* became a matter of public and religious law after the Fourth Lateran

Council first decreed its use in 1215; the Synod of Vienna subsequently reinforced its application in 1267, and Pope Paul IV supported the use of the *Judenhut* in 1555. Although the *Judenhut* later fell into disuse, local governments forced Jews to display publicly other distinguishing markers such as yellow or red badges. In some areas Jewish women were required to wear a white veil that had two blue stripes on it.[23]

As the Middle Ages in Europe gave way to the Renaissance and subsequently to the Enlightenment, Christian authorities abandoned many of these practices. In the Post-Enlightenment period, many nation-states demanded that religious subgroups conform by altering their traditional practices. In doing so, individuals were freed to make personal decisions instead of yielding to the external powers of religious authority. As Christian women began appearing in public unveiled, Jewish women faced the question of whether to assimilate by foregoing head covering or to uphold religious tradition. As Christian governments removed dress restrictions from Jews, many chose to forgo their more traditional religious costumes in favor of a more assimilated dress code. Combined with other factors, this marked the beginning of the split of Judaism into different movements based on levels of observance.

The Haskalah, or Jewish Enlightenment, took place in Europe from approximately 1770–1880. During this time period, Jews were encouraged to learn both Jewish and secular culture and language. As maskilim (Jews who were involved in the Haskalah) immersed themselves in European culture, many began to assimilate in terms of dress, language, and culture, leading to the schisms that formed modern-day progressive Judaism. A heightened understanding evolving of the dual identity of assimilated Jewry.

Historically, hair has been culturally influential in establishing a hierarchy of Jewish observance. The role of religion and assimilation proved once again to be a major concern for Jews during the three great tides of Jewish immigration to the United States—during the colonial period, between 1880–1920, and after World War II—as they found themselves geographically scattered and forced to grapple with the diasporic problem of maintaining cultural continuity within a society that held conflicting values and norms. Most Jewish women abandoned hair covering after immigrating to the United States as they struggled to assimilate into American culture or as a means of leaving pain and past behind.[24] In particular, as American hat culture declined, Jewish women were less inclined to "other" themselves through headwear.

Hats are frequently regarded as simple accessories that are subject to the whims of fashion. However, sitting on the head, hats are prominently imbued by wearer and viewer with both personal and social symbolism. They are a sign of the times and their trends mirror more than fashion—they are encoded with meaning. Since its foundation, the United States has been a hat culture. That is to say, when outside of the home—and frequently within the home—both men and women covered their heads. These hats served several purposes: they shielded the face and head from the sun, were tools of etiquette and modesty, and marked social class. Whether it was an African head wrap that symbolized Southern white power [25] or an extravagant Kentucky Derby hat, what a person wore on her head communicated volumes.

During the late nineteenth century, hat couture had reached all levels of society. Mass marketing, mail-order catalogs, and a general increase in wages and consumerism fueled an increased interest in stylish headwear. [26] Some hats marked occupational status such as identification with the military, certain sports groups, or a particular trade. In addition, practical hats still had their place, particularly among those in lower socioeconomic groups, but even the less privileged sought out stylish hats, which they used to convey refinement as well as personal character.

It was during this time period that women became increasingly involved in leisure activities. With the advent of the bicycle—and eventually the automobile—their coiffeur and headwear changed to meet their new needs. Shockingly, women adopted masculine hat styles as new fashion, including top hats for horse riding, straw sailor hats, and the derby hat (a masculine bowler renamed and marketed for women). [27]

Gender bending hats did not stop with the reappropriation of male styles. Many are quick to assume that men likely appeared bareheaded before women, but the opposite is true. As the theater and opera became affordable to the middle class, the hats of upper class women increased in size, so as to demonstrate their social standing. The only problem was that they blocked the view of those seated behind them. Unlike men who could simply remove their hats and either leave them at the coat room or hold them on their laps, women struggled to decide what to do with their hats. They were too large to check at the coat room or to hold on their laps, but, perhaps most importantly, removing their hats would ruin their hairstyles. Not only would they appear disheveled, but reattaching their hats after the show was not easily done. Women began, as early as the 1890s, appearing hatless at the theater, which marked the beginning of the end of American hat culture. [28]

Proper etiquette of the early twentieth century dictated that men and women still wear hats in order to be properly dressed. [29] As part of a consumer culture, women were interested in having numerous hats and in matching them with outfits to create ensembles. Millinery shops capitalized on this desire and promoted a feminine shopping environment that both appealed to women and encouraged them to engage in consumerism. Whether it was a hat for running errands or a hat to promenade in an Easter Parade, there was a hat for every occasion. [30]

The two World Wars created certain stumbling blocks for female hat wearers. New military headwear emerged for both men and women. These hats were part of uniforms and communicated job, rank, gender, and service.

For civilians, money was tight, supplies were limited, and women were entering the workforce. Although female hairstyles became shorter, there was no shortage of hats. As Christina Probert describes it, they were "often the one bright note among the dull clothes available."[31] In the years following World War II, hat culture began a steep downward slide. Americans were increasingly interested in informality and saw hats representing the authoritarianism and oppression against which they had been fighting.[32]

By the 1960s, hats were considered old fashioned and were relegated to formal occasions. The new political face of the United States, John F. Kennedy, publically appeared bareheaded. As the country followed the president's political leadership, they also looked to him for fashion cues. If hats were too formal for the president, they certainly were unnecessary for the common man.[33] Symbolically, getting rid of hats also indicated the American desire of mobility. Likewise, bareheadedness represented liberation from etiquette and modesty (tipping the hat or removing the hat, for example) that was in line with the cultural ideals of the time. Still, as Fiona Clark describes, ". . . in the face of this general neglect of hats most people today still choose to mark the important occasions of their lives by wearing one—this surely is evidence of how deeply rooted is the urge to dignify and decorate our heads with a hat."[34] Indeed, hats are still worn by some to weddings, religious services, or ritual events. Whether it is the bridal veil, a graduation cap, or a couture hat, ornamental headgear is still engrained in the American mindset.

Americans still wear what could be considered "practical" hats: for example, baseball caps, sun hats, tennis visors, or ski caps. However, the focus on hats as an everyday accessory has been eclipsed by hairstyling. The contemporary hair stylist is the new milliner: creating, designing, and helping women externalize their self-perception. Hatters have become increasingly fanciful by developing stunning artistic creations that are completely unwearable by the everyday woman.

Although Americans have an interest in observing the hats of British royalty, they have not widely emulated a female hat since the pill box hats worn by Jacqueline Kennedy Onassis.[35] Contemporary milliner Stephen Jones writes, "This is the magical power of a hat—its ability to reflect the character of individuals but also transform them into someone else."[36] One only needs to flip through the pages of a fashion magazine to see that Americans still seem fascinated by hats, even if they rarely wear them. Historically, Orthodox women who covered their hair with hats or scarves did not stand out when all of the women around them also wore hats. Likewise, their religious motivations were so comingled with American cultural norms that the two were sometimes indistinguishable from one another. But for contemporary Orthodox women who live outside of a hat culture, hair covering remains an externalization of their religious commitment. Hats may no longer define American social class, but they still function in terms of Jewish religious hierarchy.

For many years, it seemed as if hair covering would eventually fall into disuse as a defining marker of a pious Jewish woman. Despite the secularization and liberalization of American culture, sociologists document efforts made by religious groups to reinforce significant traditions.[37] Although greater attention has primarily focused on Christian and Muslim fundamentalism, Judaism has also experienced a less-discussed renewal. With observant families growing in size and number, as well as with the increase of *ba'alot teshuvah* (newly observant women), more Jewish women are covering their hair. The current generation of Jewish women represents cultural extremes that reflect the depth and breadth of the American Jewish experience; they have transcended a tumultuous history, endured major world wars, and survived immigration, assimilation, and enculturation. Hair covering, like those women who embrace it, has proven to be both resilient and versatile. At present, an estimated three to four percent of contemporary American Jewish women cover their hair.[38]

For these women, hair covering serves as a *siman nisuin* (sign of marriage). Hair covering signals female centered Jewish ritual and tradition. Upholding this practice emphasizes the centrality of women in preserving Orthodoxy. Hair covering serves a transitory role between the one and the many; not only does it mark a woman as married, it also marks her as part of a generation before her who made the same commitment. It represents the clearest way that an Orthodox female externally demonstrates her commitment to the protection of the group's religious values. She safeguards many private elements of practiced religion, including sexual purity laws, keeping a kosher home, and instilling Jewish education and values into children. However, her hair covering openly expresses and articulates her convictions to the secular world. The following chapters contain a study of how Jewish women apply hair covering, and their attitudes concerning their hair, exploring the ways in which the hair covering practices of a small town Orthodox synagogue struggles with the tensions of acculturation, assimilation, and identity in a context where it is difficult to live as an Orthodox Jew. Using hair covering as an entry point into the lives of these women, an understanding of the empowerment of the choice to cover (or not to cover) emerges that demonstrates the commitment of the women to safeguarding traditional Judaism. Hair covering, in this context, has become a ritualized behavior that affirms the centrality of the feminine role in the survival of Orthodoxy.

NOTES

1. To briefly summarize a religious tradition is difficult, and I do not claim to cover more than just the very basic of concepts in this introduction. Judaism is a religion rich with ritual

and spirituality. For those interested in learning more about Judaism, I suggest beginning with Stephen M. Wylen, *Settings of Silver: An Introduction to Judaism* (New York: Paulist Press, 2000). For those interested in the development of Judaism in the United States, I suggest Jonathan D. Sarna, *American Judaism: A History* (New Haven: Yale University Press, 2005). Also valuable is Hasia Diner, *The Jews of the United States, 1654–2000* (Berkeley: University of California Press, 2006).

2. The idea of being a "chosen people" for Jews does not imply a belief in superiority. Rather, Jews view chosenness as the idea that they have been chosen to be a model unto the nations. This approach places religious obligations upon Jews that are not placed upon everyone else. Likewise, as chosenness is a matter of birthright, Jews do not proselytize or seek to convert others to Judaism. Reconstructionist Jews reject the idea of chosenness, replacing it rather with a sense of vocation and service.

3. Exodus 19:3–56

4. The Abrahamic covenant is found in Genesis 12–17, which tells Abraham that he will become a great nation and that his descendants, marked by circumcision, will spread throughout the world. The Moasiac Covenant, found in Exodus 19–24, establishes Israel as a holy nation and emphasizes the importance of the Sabbath. The Israel Covenant, found in Deuteronomy 29–30, establishes the punishments for those who disobey Mosaic law and break the covenant. There are other smaller covenants which biblical scholars identify, including the Davidic Covenant (2 Samuel 7), National Covenants (Exodus 19:8, Joshua 24:24, 2 Kings 3:3, Nehemiah 10:29, Jeremiah 50:5), Isaac's Covenant (Genesis 48), Jacob's Covenant (Genesis 28), and the Noahic Covenant (Genesis 8–9).

5. Jews also rely on the Tanakh (the Hebrew Bible in its entirety), the Talmud, *halakhic* literature (including the Mishneh Torah and the Shulchan Arukh), and various kabbalistic works. Some use the word Torah to refer to the Hebrew Bible (or Old Testament) in its entirety. This is, however, misleading. The Torah, as understood here, is only the first five books of the Hebrew Bible.

6. For those interested in women's issues and the Torah, I suggest Elyse M. Goldstein's *The Women's Torah Commentary*. Also an excellent resource is Elle Frankel's *Five Books of Miriam: A Woman's Commentary on the Torah*. An excellent biblical resource is Carol Meyers, Toni Craven, and Ross Shephard Kraemer's *Women in Scripture: A Dictionary of Named and Unnamed Women in the Bible, the Apocrypha/Deuterocanonical Books, and the New Testament*. Finally, standard to all of feminist biblical commentary is Carol A. Newsom and Sharon H. Ringe's *Women's Bible Commentary*.

7. Genesis 2:1–3, Exodus 16:26, Exodus 20:8–11

8. An essential read for those interested in the Sabbath and Jewish spirituality is Abraham Joshua Heschel *The Sabbath* (New York: Farrar Straus Giroux, 2005). A practical guide for those concerned about how to merge Sabbath observance with modern life is Meredith Jacobs, *The Modern Jewish Mom's Guide to Shabbat; Connect and Celebrate—Bring Your Family Together with the Friday Night Meal* New York: Harper Books, 2007).

9. A good reference for those interested in kosher dietary laws is Lise Stern, *How to Keep Kosher: A Comprehensive Guide to Understanding Jewish Dietary Laws* New York: William Morrow, 2004). Stern considers what it means to keep kosher on a multitude of levels and focuses on the spirituality of the practice as well as the practicalities.

10. Consult Sarna's *American Judaism* for more on the actual evolution of the various movements, their development, the politics involved in their division, and the impact that it has had on American Jewish culture.

11. The Orthodox Union and the National Council of Young Israel do provide some leadership, but their authority is not universally accepted, nor do all Orthodox congregations recognize their authority.

12. See Jeffrey S. Gurock, *Orthodox Jews in America* (Bloomington: Indiana University Press, 2009).

13. See Samuel Heilman, *Sliding to the Right: The Contest for the Future of American Jewish Orthodoxy* (Berkeley: University of California Press, 2006).

14. See Samuel Heilman and Steven Cohen, *Cosmopolitans and Parochials: Modern Orthodox Jews in America* (Chicago: University of Chicago Press, 1999).

15. See Samuel Heilman, *Defenders of the Faith: Inside Ultra-Orthodox Jewry* (Berkley: University of California Press, 1999).

16. See Jerome Mintz, *Hasidic People: A Place in the New World* (Cambridge, MA: Harvard University Press, 1998).

17. See Neil Gillman, *Conservative Judaism: The New Century* (New York: Behrman, 1993).

18. See Rebecca Alpert and Jacob Staub, *Exploring Judaism: A Reconstructionist Approach* (New York: The Reconstructionist Press, 2000).

19. See Dana Evan Kaplan, *American Reform Judaism: An Introduction* (New Brunswick: NJ: Rutgers University Press, 2003).

20. The Bible is understood, for the purposes of this paper, to be the Hebrew Bible. Plain Christian women and some Christian fundamentalist women practice hair covering based on the New Testament text found in I Corinthians 11:2–16.

21. Kelly Olson, *Dress and the Roman Woman: Self Presentation and Society* (New York: Routledge, 2008), 20–25.

22. Judith Baskin, "Jewish Women in the Middle Ages," in *Jewish Women in Historical Perspective, ed. Judith Baskin (Detroit: Wayne State University Press, 1991)*, 101–27.

23. Johann Maier, *Geschichte der jüdischen Religion: Von der Zeit Alexander des Grossen bis zur Aufklärung mit einem Ausblick of das 19./20. Jahrhundert* (Frankfurt, Germany: De Gruyter, 1972), 28.

24. Jenna Weissman Joselit, *The Wonders of America: Reinventing Jewish Culture 1880–1950* (New York: Picado, 2002).

25. Helen Bradley Griebel, "The African American Woman's Headwrap: Unwinding the Symbols," in *Dress and Identity*, ed. Mary Ellen Roach-Higgens, Joanne B. Eicher, and Kim K. P. Johnson (New York: Capital Cities Media, 1995), 445–60. Griebel does not address the evolution of the African American headwrap as symbolic of black power. Her work, however, creates a foundation for interpreting encoded messages in the practice.

26. Madeline Ginsburg, *The Hat: Trends and Traditions* (New York: Barrons, 1990).

27. Diana Crane, *Fashion and Its Social Agendas: Class, Gender, and Identity in Clothing* (Chicago: University of Chicago Press, 2000), 103–18.

28. Neil Steinberg, *Hatless Jack: The President, the Fedora, and the History of American Style* (New York: Plume, 2004), 245–47.

29. Christina Probert, *Hats in Vogue Since 1910* (New York: Abbeville Press, 1981), 8.

30. Colin McDowell, *Hats: Status, Style, and Glamour* (New York: Rizzoli, 1992), 104–105.

31. Probert, *Hats in Vogue*, 58.

32. Ginsburg, *The Hat*, 123–24.

33. See Steinberg, *Hatless Jack*.

34. Fiona Clark, *Hats* (New York: Quite Specific Media Group, 1984), 7.

35. Ginsburg, *The Hat*, 132.

36. Stephen Jones, *Hats: An Anthology* (London: V & A Publishing, 2009), 14.

37. See Reynolds, *Plain Women*; Dean M. Kelley, *Why Conservative Churches are Growing: A Study in Sociology of Religion* (Macon, GA: Mercer University Press 1996).

38. Diane Simon *Hair: Public, Political, Extremely Personal* (New York: St. Martin's Press, 2001), 162.

Chapter Three

Splitting Hairs

*The Struggle for Community Definition in a
Small Town Orthodox Synagogue*

Few local Lancaster County, Pennsylvania, residents know where Degel Israel Synagogue is located. Those that do usually only know the building because of the Sunday evening bingo group that rents the auditorium. Others confuse it with Shaarai Shomayim, the local Reform Synagogue—a mistake I usually recognize when the speaker describes the façade of the building as striking or beautiful. Degel Israel sits tucked behind large overgrown trees along a busy road on the outskirts of downtown Lancaster. From the outside, the building is unimpressive—ivy covers the white stucco walls, and the building appears empty. The sanctuary's stunning stained glass windows are not visible from the road. Not only are Lancaster County residents unfamiliar with its location, but they generally express a disbelief that Orthodox Jews even live in the area. Yet despite all odds, nestled in the heart of Amish country, a small and faithful Orthodox synagogue perseveres.

The perceptive eye will notice traces of the local Orthodox presence. There are more obvious examples: caftan clad men with white knee socks and flowing *payot* making their way to Sabbath services on foot or tents erected during Sukkot. Other examples are less obvious: the Tuesday morning flurry at the meat counter at one local grocery store that special orders kosher meat or house lights left on all night during the Sabbath. Is Lancaster's Orthodox population ignored because it is so assimilated that no one notices them or because there are so few of them? The reality of the lived experience of Lancaster's Orthodox Jews rests somewhere in between these two extremes.

CREATING THE FOUNDATION: AN OVERVIEW OF
AMERICAN ORTHODOXY

In this chapter I will begin by offering a demographic overview of contemporary American Orthodoxy. This will serve as a foundation for understanding the ways in which Degel Israel is both typical and atypical. I will then offer a concise overview of the history and current demographics of Orthodoxy in Lancaster County, Pennsylvania, including a discussion of American small community Jewry. Finally, my analysis will address questions of how Degel Israel has developed coping mechanisms such as an acceptance of a diversity of observance or in the ways in which they have repackaged and marketed the synagogue. This analysis culminates with the argument that it is the central role of Jewish women in the Lancaster community that has ensured the survival of Lancaster's Orthodox Jews.

Unlike other conservative religious groups—for example the Amish, the Hutterites, or Old Order Mennonites—Orthodox Jews are not a rurally based group. Likewise, although there is a certain sense of living counterculturally, their lifestyles are highly assimilated and modern. They are employed by and interact with the local community, have attended secular colleges and graduate schools, and are fully assimilated in terms of technology. Many even appear assimilated in terms of dress or head/hair covering. Even Orthodox Jews who wear more traditional dress embody a paradox of modernity with their cell phones holstered at their hips. They defy typical patterns of acculturation and have created and maintained a careful balance of assimilation and counterculturalism. They are, in many ways, a living contradiction.

American Jews are primarily urban dwellers who have largely settled the Northeast. Indeed, the most recent National Jewish Population Survey finds that 43 percent of American Jews live in the Northeast, with New York being the top metropolitan area, boasting an estimated 24 percent of the country's Jews.[1] This is a significant drop from the 1960 survey, which found 67 percent of American Jews living in the Northeast.[2] This shift seems largely to do with the increase of Jews in the South, in particular South Florida, which now boasts 8 percent of the national Jewish population.[3] Not only is this typical of other American migration patterns,[4] but it is indicative of the trend of older Jews retiring to warmer climates. Indeed, the South is home to the largest population of Jews over the age of 65,[5] (with more than half living in South Florida.[6]

American Jews living in the Northeast have an average household size of 2.4 persons and possess the highest levels of education among American Jews. Sixty-four percent of northeastern Jews over the age of 25 have completed college, and 31 percent have completed a graduate degree. Not surprisingly they also earn the highest median household income ($59,800). Of American Jews, they are the least likely to own their own homes—only 60 percent have purchased their homes,[7] which is not surprising given the propensity to rent in large urban cities like New York, Philadelphia, Boston, and Baltimore.

Religiously, the Northeast is also home to the majority of Orthodox Jews. Twelve percent of northeastern Jews classify themselves as Orthodox, which is significantly higher than elsewhere in the country.[8] Those who live in the New York metropolitan area are even more likely to self-identify as Orthodox; Orthodox Jews compose 17 percent of all Jews in the greater New York area.[9] Although these numbers may not, at first glance, seem like a significant portion of the Jewish population, consider that 68 percent of American Orthodox Jews find their home in the Northeast.[10] Not surprisingly, northeastern Jews, particularly those in the New York metropolitan area, are also more likely than their national counterparts to light Chanukkah candles, hang a Mezuzah, fast on Yom Kippur, light Sabbath candles, and keep a kosher home. They are also the most likely to attend services at least once a month.[11] This increase in ritual observance is likely partially bolstered by the local Orthodox population. Indeed, 78 percent of Orthodox Jews refrain from all forms of work on the Sabbath; 75 percent keep fully kosher outside of the home; 86 percent maintain a fully kosher kitchen; and nearly 60 percent attend religious services at least once a week.[12]

American Orthodox Jews, who make up 10 percent of the general Jewish population,[13] number approximately 529,000 individuals with 324,000 adults and 205,000 children under the age of eighteen.[14] They also boast a high synagogue membership rate. 46 percent of American Jews belong to a synagogue, and 21 percent belong to an Orthodox synagogue.[15]

The Orthodox community must face issues of retention. Forty-one percent of Orthodox Jews who were raised within Orthodoxy continue to identify with the group.[16] The majority of those leaving Orthodoxy still consider themselves Jewish,[17] with the most common realignment being with Conservative Judaism.[18] Only one out of every five Orthodox Jews was raised in another Jewish denomination, with the majority moving from Conservative to Orthodox.[19]

Unlike other small religious groups who fear the impact of aging congregations, Orthodox Jews are surprisingly young. Nationally the largest percentage (34 percent) of the Orthodox population is between 18–34 years old. In fact, 88 percent of the Orthodox population is under the age of 65.[20] This includes a significantly higher percentage of Orthodox youth under the age of 18, due, in large part, to the high birthrate of the Orthodox community.

The average American birth rate is 2.1 children per household.[21] American Jews have a lower average birthrate of 1.86 children. However, the typical Modern Orthodox family has 3.3 children; ultraorthodox families average 6.6 children; and Hasidic couples have an astounding average of 7.9 children.[22] This figure for Orthodox families is significantly different from the general Jewish population, which has a higher proportion of seniors and a lower population of children.[23]

When considering the choices being made by such a young population, commitment to Orthodoxy by youth can be seen through their marriage and educational choices. First, they are choosing, much more so than their more liberal Jewish counterparts, to marry endogamously. Only 5 percent of the Orthodox population married non-Jews between 1996 and 2001, which is down from 10 percent in 1985–1990. When compared to the 47 percent of American Jews who intermarry, the Orthodox priority of endogamous marriage is apparent.[24] The children produced of these marriages are also extremely likely to attend a private Orthodox day school. Day school attendance continues to increase, which is especially apparent when considering that only 18 percent of those over the age of 75 attended an Orthodox day school, in contrast with 91 percent of current Orthodox children who are receiving such education.[25]

Taken together, the data suggest that the archetypal American Jew would live in the Northeast, most likely the New York metropolitan area. She would be well educated and most likely self-identify as Reform. If she were Orthodox, she would likely be young, married, day school educated, and have a higher number of children than her Reform sisters. This begs the question, just how "normal" is the tiny Orthodox community in Lancaster, Pennsylvania? Demographically there may be similarities, but the lived experiences of Lancaster's Orthodox community are drastically different from most of American Orthodoxy.

ORTHODOXY IN AMISH COUNTRY

Degel Israel Synagogue is an Orthodox congregation located in Lancaster, Pennsylvania. The synagogue, situated in the heart of Amish country, is distinctive. Historically, Lancaster was home to the first Jewish community in central Pennsylvania. In fact, it is as one of the few cities in the United States that was home to a pre-Revolutionary War Jewish settlement beginning as early as 1747.[26] However, unlike Harrisburg and York, Pennsylvania, it is no longer an area associated with having a Jewish, especially Orthodox, population. With approximately 508,000 residents, Lancaster County is home to about 6.0 percent of the state's population. The area is predominantly white (93.2 percent) and American-born (96.8 percent).[27] The city of Lancaster is more racially diverse, with only 61.6 percent of residents identifying as white but with most other demographics remaining quite similar.[28] The most recent Lancaster County statistics on religious organizations identify 470,658 individuals who affiliate with a particular religion—about 93.0 percent of the total population. Approximately 5,000 are considered "Other," including those who identify as Baha'i, Church of Jesus Christ of Latter-day Saints, Hindu, Jewish, Muslim, and Unitarian Universalist.[29]

Lancaster County is not only predominantly white—it is also overwhelmingly Christian. With almost 90,000 Evangelical Protestants and an equal number of Mainline Protestants, coupled with nearly 50,000 Catholics and over 240,000 other self-identifying Christians, 92.0 percent of the local population identifies as Christian, which is about 10 percent above the national average.[30] Members of the three local synagogues are certainly in the minority.

With between 6.0 and 6.4 million Jews in the United States (about 1.7 percent of the total population),[31] approximately 295,000 Jews live in Pennsylvania,[32] making up 2.3 percent of the state's population.[33] There are an estimated 3,000 Jews living in the Lancaster area,[34] comprising only 0.59 percent of the local population. There is reason to believe, however, that this number is significantly inflated. According to telephone queries on January 10, 2011, the local Reform congregation reported a membership of 353, and the local Conservative synagogue identified 158 current members. This inflated number could be caused by non-practicing Jews who still identified themselves as Jewish on the survey or by including non-local college students.

It is difficult to calculate an exact membership for Degel Israel. Around 80 families pay for membership at the synagogue. In this system, an individual as well as a family of four is counted as a single unit. Further complicating this count is that some of those families do not attend the synagogue and hold membership elsewhere. They maintain membership to honor a historic family affiliation, as a means of supporting a struggling congregation, or as a sign of solidarity. Some local Conservative Jews hold dual membership in order to send their children to Degel Israel's Hebrew school, as the Conservative Hebrew school is extremely small. Saturday morning Sabbath services typically garner between ten to twenty men and five to ten women, about 1.0 percent of local Jewry and 0.005 percent of the general local population.

That Degel Israel is in the Northeast is no surprise, but it fails to conform to the general trends of Jewish urbanization. Contemporary American Jews, as a whole, are city dwellers.[35] This trend toward living in cities is especially true of the Orthodox.[36] Those living in suburbia or in isolated communities are forced to contend with the difficult dynamic of balancing community integration, traditionalism, and spiritual cohesion. Those Jews living in suburbia generally live in rather homogenous religious communities where, as Etan Diamond describes it, they share "backgrounds, attitudes, and lifestyles [which] create a sense of community among congregational members, who look out for one another, offering help in times of need and a smile in times of happiness."[37] This homogeneity is, however, not the case of Degel Israel.

Located an hour north of Baltimore and two hours west of Philadelphia, Degel Israel has become home to what can only be described as a mixed group of Orthodoxy. Were the same individuals to live in a different location, they surely would have subdivided into separate synagogues based on levels of observance and religious belief. Geographic isolation has, however, brought them together under one roof. Although other small and struggling Orthodox synagogues might compromise and merge with Conservative synagogues, Degel Israel's members have resisted this change. Their self-identification as Orthodox is strongly associated with their traditional worship style. In fact, some promotional pieces and newsletters have proclaimed Degel Israel as "Lancaster's Traditional Synagogue." Although levels of home observance vary within Degel Israel's membership, services have a commonly accepted structure: gender segregated seating, only men at the *bimah* (altar), modest dress, a fully Hebrew liturgy, and traditional interpretations of the text. They may accept a variety of Orthodox observance, but their shared identity is decidedly more conservative and traditional than the local Conservative synagogue. Despite their differences, they are wholly dependent on each other if they wish to have a local Orthodox community.

Unlike the Jews of Harrisburg, Pennsylvania, and other suburban Orthodox populations who maintain a distinct Jewish neighborhood, Lancaster's Orthodoxy is spread not only around the city but also the county. Most members of the local Orthodox population own their homes. Only the most observant, about ten families, live within walking distance to the synagogue. Because of this geographic scattering and lack of a distinct Orthodox neighborhood, most of Degel Israel's members are the only Orthodox Jews, and sometimes the only Jews, in their neighborhoods. Their Jewish community, then, must entirely revolve around the actual synagogue.

Members of Degel Israel are in Lancaster County for two reasons: either they were born into the community or relocated to the area for employment. It is generally the older members of the community who were born in the area and have remained in Lancaster County to raise their families and ultimately retire. Younger and middle aged couples are more likely to have relocated to the area for employment or, in a few cases, educational opportunities. There is no one particular company or job type that has especially drawn Orthodoxy to the area. Rather, the congregants of Degel Israel are employed in a wide array of positions. Men in the congregation, for example, teach at local colleges, oversee the koshering process at local farms and agricultural packaging plants, run a highly profitable telecommunications firm, work in television production, oversee kosher meals at campus cafeterias, work in military recruitment, serve in the rabbinate, and work as accountants, doctors, and lawyers. Women are employed as lawyers, teachers, in retail, optometry, informational technology, nursing, and a variety of other fields. In addition, residency programs at local hospitals and a prestigious watch making program run by Rolex also bring congregants to the area.

Ranging from members of the Belz Hasidim to Modern Orthodox families who are not *shomer shabbos* (those who strictly observe Sabbath laws), it is hard to imagine a more diverse congregation. One only needs to take a quick glance into the sanctuary on Saturday mornings to be made aware of the striking diversity in terms of observance. Rather than seeing similarly clad individuals *davening* (praying) together, the men's section ranges from fur *shtreimels* (fur hats worn by Hasidic men) and caftans with knee socks to baseball caps and jeans. The women's appearances range from *frum* (religiously devout) with completely covered hair and long dresses covering the ankles to short sleeved dresses with free flowing locks. It is, however, only through the acceptance of such a diverse membership that Degel Israel is able to persist, forcing members to deal with these tensions in light of maintaining a shared community identity.

THE REPACKAGING OF ORTHODOXY IN LANCASTER

The geographic location of Degel Israel has a significant impact on its Orthodox community. Urban Jews may exist as a minority in the United States, but the Orthodox community in Lancaster exists as an extreme minority. Their life experiences are profoundly different than their urban counterparts. If we accept that their lifestyles vary from urban Jewish communities, how are their lives similar or different than other Jews living in small communities?

The National Jewish Population Survey identifies forty large metropolitan areas where Jews are concentrated. Jews living outside of these areas are considered to live in "small communities."[38] An estimated 802,000 Jews live in small communities, equaling 15 percent of American Jewry.[39] This sector of the Jewish population is less likely to be "Jewishly connected" and significantly more likely to be intermarried or cohabitating with non-Jews.[40] Demographically, small communities are younger and have significantly lower numbers of children.[41] Only half of the children raised in small communities are even being raised to self-identify as Jewish.[42] Levels of Jewish education for those children who are being raised as Jews in small communities are also drastically lower. Those who receive religious education are educated through synagogues or Jewish Community Center programming and not religious day schools. Indeed, urban Jewish youth are three times more likely to attend a Jewish day school than their nonurban counterparts.[43]

In terms of religious observance, small community Jews are less likely to host or attend a Passover Seder, light Chanukkah candles, fast on Yom Kippur, or keep a kosher kitchen.[44] Although synagogue attendance rates are similar,[45] Jews in small communities are more likely to say that their participation in Jewish activities has decreased in the last five years.[46] Not surprisingly, small community Jews report lower rates of feeling "a strong sense of belonging to the Jewish people" and are less likely to say "that being Jewish is very important in their lives."[47]

When considering small Jewish communities, it is crucial to understand how few Orthodox Jews live outside of metropolitan areas. Nonurban Jews are most likely to self-identify as Reform, "Just Jewish," or secular. Synagogue membership follows similar patterns.[48]

With only 3 percent of small community Jews identifying as Orthodox and such a high number identifying as "Just Jewish" or secular, it is not surprising that levels of observance in such communities are substantially lower than major metropolitan areas. It is also not surprising that so little inquiry into small community Orthodox behaviors and beliefs has taken place. 3 percent of the total small Jewish community population equates to only 24,060 individuals, roughly 0.37 percent of the total American Jewish population and 0.007 percent of the total general population. Small community Orthodoxy represents a tiny fragment of American religion—one that, by all calculations, should have assimilated and disappeared long ago.

The 80 families of Degel Israel exist on the periphery of both their general community and the national and local Jewish community. They seem to be in a prime position to assimilate and move away from Orthodoxy. What factors function to undergird their Orthodox affiliation? The survival of Lancaster's Orthodox community stems from two primary responses to acculturation: their adaptation to multiple levels of observance and their efforts to be forward thinking and innovative.

Before I visited services at Degel Israel for the first time, I met with the Rabbi to discuss the Lancaster *eruv* (a ritual enclosure or fence around a home or community that allows for the carrying of objects during the Sabbath). Our conversation included discussion of the local Jewish community, and I expressed uncertainty about the congregation's level of observance. When he did not comment on my remarks, I was unsure of what to expect when I attended services the following week. Local Reform and Conservative Jewish friends had made comments that led me to believe that the congregation was extremely observant, comprised largely of ultraorthodox members. These forewarnings, although well intentioned, were completely false and belie Lancaster's nonorthodox Jews' unfamiliarity with the group. My notes reflecting on my first visit indicate the confusion I felt in terms of classifying the congregation. I wrote, "Not like other Orthodox *shuls* I've visited. Were there visitors there this week or are they really so diverse? There was a guy in a baseball cap sitting rows behind a Hasid. Not at all what I expected!"

My first impressions of the diversity of Degel Israel were largely based on dress. I recognized that this did not necessarily imply levels of observance or, as Solomon Poll suggests, social stratification.[49] In this case it served to indicate a lack of the homogeneity that one expects in Orthodox synagogues. Clearly this congregation cannot be labeled or associated with one particular branch of Orthodoxy. Looking beneath the surface, I was left to wonder if there was an expected level of observance or belief.

As I became increasingly familiar with the community, it was apparent that the synagogue houses a variety of observance and belief. I have been invited by a synagogue member to go for coffee on a minor fasting holiday; on the other hand, I have also observed children deny a drink of water until an appropriate cup could be found in the home of a family who maintained a kosher kitchen—their level of *kashrut*, however, was not to the standards of the children's family. Clearly, there is no general consensus for observance. What these anecdotes demonstrate is that despite their differences, somehow congregants have established a shared middle ground that functions as the basis of their community. This commonality is twofold: a shared community identification and the actual Sabbath service.

The defining factor that establishes congregants' community identity is their shared understanding that they are "other." This othering takes place on two levels: first, as Orthodox Jews, they identify themselves as clearly different from Reform or Conservative Jews. This is an important distinction for them, especially in terms of worship style and lifestyle choices. Second, they are decidedly different from the greater Lancaster community. This type of subcultural identification is not unfamiliar for the area but countercultural religious identification is typically associated with local Anabaptists or evangelical Christians.

Their desire to foster a strong sense of community identity is not surprising. In fact, it functions as a survival tactic. If they do not create a strong group bond and barrier, they risk total assimilation. They are familiar with the plight and frequent demise of other small Orthodox communities. They have a clear vision of their destiny if they do not create a cohesive unit. They must shield themselves not only from the dangers of general American acculturation, but also from the pressures to conform to the local nonorthodox Jewish population. Although they may not practice the same level of home observance, their commonality is that they are consciously not affiliated with other branches of Judaism and consider their lifestyle decidedly Jewish.

The primary way through which they demonstrate their shared commitment to Orthodox Judaism is the actual Sabbath service. Regardless of their home practice, the service functions as a shared community based event. They accept certain aspects of the service structure and the interpretation of the biblical texts in sermons, thereby creating a cultural scene in which they participate and with which they identify. Celebrating the Sabbath together includes the actual services as well as shared meals, textual study, and socialization. Unlike other synagogues where the entire Sabbath experience lasts less than two hours, if one fully participates in the complete Degel Israel Sabbath experience, an entire Saturday is quickly spent alternating between services, food, ritual, social time, and text study.

Without this weekly event that forces social bonding, the community would struggle to remain cohesive. Unlike other Orthodox communities in which congregants live in the same neighborhood and interact socially with one another throughout the week, Degel Israel comes together at Sabbath services. The importance of this shared community time in light of geographic dispersion can be clearly seen in the synagogue's parking lot. Parked directly behind the building during the Sabbath are campers—usually at least one, sometimes several. Members who are *shomer shabbos* but do not live within walking distance have purchased campers and literally sleep in the parking lot. Others have rented nearby apartments for use during the Sabbath. Those who cannot afford to do so and still refrain from traveling on the Sabbath are confined to their homes. One family, who oversees kosher packaging at a local farm, expresses an extreme feeling of disconnection. Without children in the Hebrew school, unable to attend Sabbath services, and with farming work conflicts prohibiting them from attending many social events, they feel like they exist outside of the community. The life of an Orthodox Jew in Lancaster County can be extremely isolating. The Sabbath service is the key way that community identification is formed and maintained.

Despite their variety of dress, congregants know upon entering Degel Israel that it is an Orthodox synagogue. The *mechitza* (a partition that separates men and women in the sanctuary) is prominent and creates gender-segregated seating. Only men are invited to chant from the *bimah*. All of the men have their heads covered in some form. The majority of them are wrapped in *tallisim* (prayer shawls). The Hebrew liturgy is familiar and repeated each week from *Siddurim* (prayer books) that are without transliteration and, if they have English translation, with traditional renderings of the liturgical texts.

In some ways worshipping at Degel Israel is like stepping back in time. The traditional *davening* styles, the familiar liturgy, and the reliance on Hebrew hearkens back to the Great Wave of Immigration (1880–1920), when most Orthodox immigrants from Eastern Europe established synagogues resembling their Old World roots. However, outsiders should not assume that the congregation has not adapted to the times. Indeed, in addition to a shared commitment to community and traditional worship styles, Degel Israel is committed to a progressive stance toward Orthodox practice and belief. There are three primary ways in which Degel Israel members are innovative: through their efforts to repackage themselves and attract transplants to the area, in their development of unique educational opportunities, and in their willingness to compromise internally on certain issues of practice.

Synagogue members have recognized that without growth, they will eventually die out. Not only do they need to grow in order to replace deceased membership, but they must also account for general membership loss either through relocation (usually to Baltimore) or through lack of Orthodox self-identification.[50] The simple solution is, of course, to attract new families to settle in the area. The great difficulty, however, is making Lancaster County attractive to urban Orthodoxy.

The congregation acknowledges that there are certain conditions that they cannot change. For example, families will need to commute long distances to take their children to Orthodox day schools until the community is large enough to finance their own. However, they identified three key stumbling blocks that they could overcome in order to repackage their community and make it more attractive: the *mechitza*, the *eruv*, and the *mikveh*. Through a concentrated and nationwide fundraising effort, they were first able to raise enough funds to refurbish and modernize their *mechitza*. This was followed by the creation of a *mikveh*, much to the relief of several women who had previously been forced to commute nearly an hour to Harrisburg, Pennsylvania, in order to use another congregation's *mikveh*. The last step in their repackaging of their community was the construction of an *eruv*. This final project was an extremely costly and intensely bureaucratic process which took years to complete.

Although the *mechitza* was a onetime investment, both the *mikveh* and the *eruv* require constant fundraising and community volunteerism in order to be maintained. Why would a community with so few *shomer shabbos* members and relatively few women who use the *mikveh* invest so much time, effort, and money into two things that have not drastically changed their quality of life? The answer from Degel Israel members almost always comes in the form of the oft-quoted line from the popular movie *Field of Dreams* (1989), "If you build it, they will come."[51] They have changed the deterrents that they have control over, even offering to help with relocation costs and job placement. The only thing they are unable to change, and perhaps the largest hurdle, is their geographic location.

One creative way that they have negotiated the difficulty of living in Lancaster County is through the establishment of the Lancaster Yeshiva Center. This institution of Jewish learning is unique to Degel Israel, because it is the only American *yeshiva* that blends Jewish learning with trade training. In other words, it is a vocational institution in which the young men spend half of each day studying Jewish texts and the other half learning a craft, such as carpentry, painting, or masonry. Their career training is never in competition with their Orthodox lifestyle. As their mission statement clarifies, "The goal of the Lancaster Yeshiva Center is to teach a trade within the framework of Torah, empowering our students to be *ehrlich*, contributing members of society."[52]

Degel Israel is in a unique position to offer such a program. Unlike urban centers, its rural geography affords a better location for trade training. This training fills a special need for the larger American Orthodox community—the need for vocational training alongside full-time Jewish learning for men. Whether it is because the young men in the program are not capable of intense higher learning or because they are simply not interested, they would have difficulty receiving such vocational training elsewhere. Typical apprenticeships would conflict with their Orthodox lifestyle whether it is time for prayers, observing the Sabbath, the availability of kosher food, or the celebration of Jewish holidays.

One might wonder why such a small community would undertake such a large venture. True to their motto, "Torah and Trade," the Lancaster Yeshiva Center has much to offer to its young men, but, perhaps most importantly, it has also solved two key problems for Degel Israel. First, the male students live in communal housing behind the synagogue and are required to attend morning prayers. This ensures that there is always a *minyan* (the quorum of ten men required for certain religious events and rituals). Second, their tuition also helps to support the community financially.

Their presence in the community has also had two unintentional results. First, as the young men put their skills to work, each year they refurbish a rundown home in the heart of Lancaster City. This house is later given or sold at a very low cost to a deserving member of the local Lancaster community. This has created a sense of local involvement and identity. Unlike the Amish or Old Order Mennonites of the area, who also often work as tradesmen and are perceived as uninterested in downtown Lancaster, the Lancaster Yeshiva Center's projects are usually in the worst neighborhoods of Lancaster. Their hard work and renovated house are an investment in the community and helps to build bridges between Degel Israel and Lancaster's residents. This type of community ownership helps to avoid some of the racial and religious tensions felt in other communities as Orthodoxy struggles to integrate and coexist with its neighbors.[53]

The other unintentional impact of the Lancaster Yeshiva Center is the interconnectedness that it fosters between Degel Israel and other Orthodox communities. In other words, it puts Degel Israel on the map. Upon graduating the program, most of the young men return to their home congregations. However, after a successful time at the Lancaster Yeshiva Center, the young man's home congregation is more likely to send additional students or even monetary support to Degel Israel. These connections can be lifelines for the Lancaster community, whether it is for financial reasons or, more often, matchmaking or job placement.

The innovative thinking and creative spirit of the congregation is obvious in their development of the Lancaster Yeshiva Center. This type of creative problem solving can also be observed in their own intrasynagogue compromises. In order to retain membership, they have had to collectively agree to accept certain things that would surely have caused a schism in other synagogues. Perhaps the clearest example of this is the bat mitzvah. Although there are some progressive Orthodox Jews who bat mitzvah their daughters, Orthodoxy remains, at large, uninvolved in this rite of passage.[54] Certain families at Degel Israel, particularly those who also hold membership at the local Conservative congregation, felt strongly that they wanted to bat mitzvah their daughters. Unsurprisingly, this request was met with great debate.

Ultimately the congregation reached a middle ground. The young woman studies with the Rabbi and prepares in the same way that young men do. On the actual day of her bat mitzvah, however, she is not called to the *bimah* to chant her Torah portion. Rather, she offers a bat mitzvah speech in the assembly room during *Kiddush* (the blessing said over wine during the Sabbath and Jewish holidays) after the service. At her private family events later in the day, she has the opportunity to chant her Torah portion. These events are typically attended by members of the congregation, including the Rabbi and Rebbetzin. However, because they occur outside of the synagogue services, members who are uncomfortable with the idea of a bat mitzvah do not attend.

This compromise was long in the making. The congregation tried several different arrangements until this practice was developed.[55] This type of adaptation and change is what allows Degel Israel to function—without flexibility, the congregation would splinter into such tiny fragments that it would collapse.

A WOMAN'S WORK IS NEVER DONE

Degel Israel adheres to the Orthodox conventions of having a male rabbi and restricting women from leading services or reading from the Torah. Such decisions have led many scholars to describe Jewish religious structure as patriarchal. However, although outsiders are quick to critique Orthodoxy as steeped in patriarchy, all of the aforementioned ways in which Degel Israel has repackaged and redefined itself hinge on women's issues.

First, the general repackaging of the synagogue to make it more appealing for transplants to the area entirely is centered on women. The establishment of a *mikveh* is, of course, the most overt example. However, the creating of the new *mechitza* is also something that the female congregants identified as critical. One might assume that a *mechitza's* purpose is to discourage women's participation, because of its function of gender segregation during services. However, the new *mechitza* at Degel Israel has a Plexiglas back wall, allowing the women who sit there to feel more fully included in the services. They have chosen to worship in a synagogue that has gender segregated seating—which is crucial to the traditional identity with which they associate—but they wish to have the choice of where to sit. They may either choose to sit on the sides of the sanctuary, where they are fully segregated from the men, or they may sit at the back, where they have a full "unobstructed" view of the entire sanctuary. Synagogue leadership believes that by offering this choice, female newcomers will be more likely to feel comfortable, because they can select their seat according to their level of observance.

The establishment of an *eruv* in Lancaster was also motivated by the concerns of female congregants. Although it benefits all *shomer shabbos* members, it is the women who most greatly feel its impact. Through its institution, they are able to push baby carriages, carry young children, and tote diapers, bottles, or other necessary childcare items with them during the Sabbath. With the inclusion of a local park within the *eruv*, they also have the option of taking their children there during the Sabbath, which helps to foster an increased sense of community through social opportunities. In short, the *eruv* allows young mothers to participate in services—something which would be denied to them if the *eruv* did not exist. Because Degel Israel is especially interested in attracting young families to the region, the *eruv* was the most important implementation of their repackaging plan.

Even the Lancaster Yeshiva Center has had a significant impact on the women of Degel Israel. It was through the women's hard work and effort that the initial classes of young men survived the program. They prepared three meals a day to serve to the students—an act that frequently could not be prepared at home. The families of Degel Israel do not all maintain the same level of *kashrut*—because of this, most of these meals could not be prepared ahead of time. Instead, the women had to purchase the ingredients and prepare them in the synagogue's kitchen. With the addition of limited kitchen space in the dormitory, the young men are able to prepare their own breakfast and lunch. However, the women still prepare a nightly warm dinner.

Beneath these more overt examples of women's issues at Degel Israel is the reliance on the women for the synagogue's continuity. Without the tireless efforts of the female membership, life as an Orthodox Jew in Lancaster would be impossible. There are three main ways in which this plays out: in the procurement and preparation of food, in the educational choices for their children, and in the amount of community volunteerism.

Since the beginning of my time at Degel Israel, I am acutely aware each time I go to the grocery store of how easy it is for me to do my weekly food shopping. I have made several trips to Baltimore with synagogue members—either riding along or after being persuaded to take senior members out for a "short ride" to pick up a few "necessities." It takes about three hours total, round trip, to drive to Baltimore, but the magic of Reisterstown Road is undeniable. Crammed within about a mile stretch of busy city road is every possible kosher option: butchers, bakeries, grocers, delis, wine stores, confectionaries, bagel places, Dunkin' Donuts, Subway, Japanese and Chinese restaurants, and, perhaps most importantly, pizza.

The first time I visited a kosher pizza restaurant with one of my Lancaster Orthodox friends, I ordered one slice of pizza. She ordered four pies. I thought she had misspoken at first, but she had not. She purchased two pies for a friend and two that she would freeze herself for nights when she was feeling pressed for time and needed a quick dinner option. Life without takeout food options can certainly be tough on a working mother.[56]

More often than not, the women make these shopping trips alone. However, senior members who no longer drive rely on the kindness of their Orthodox sisters. Often this translates into a shopping list given to a younger woman who is making the trip. Sometimes, though, it means carpooling. These shared car rides can be tricky. Careful calculation goes not only into how many seats are needed, but, more importantly, how much cargo space will be necessary. As I learned the hard way (in an event that resulted in several older women having to unhappily ride with shopping bags on their laps), a car trunk fills quickly when one cannot do regular local grocery shopping.

I share these anecdotes as a means of demonstrating how reliant the women are on one another and, additionally, how their careful food procurement and preparation is to the community at large. It would be one thing if these women all were homemakers, but it is taken to another level when one considers that most work a full time job and still must drive to Baltimore to do the bulk of their grocery shopping.[57]

For mothers of school aged children, these grocery shopping trips to Baltimore can sometimes be combined with their school carpool. If they wish to send their children to an Orthodox day school, they have two options: they can commute to Harrisburg, Pennsylvania, to a program that runs until the eighth grade, or they can take their children to Baltimore. Almost all of the families at Degel Israel choose Baltimore generally because they feel the program is more traditional and partly because of the need to be able to drive both younger and older children in the same direction.

The day school system helps to ensure several things for parents. First, it encourages a strong sense of Orthodox self-identification. Not only does it shelter children from outside influences, but it also affords them a sense of normality. When surrounded by other Orthodox youth, their family's lifestyle choices and beliefs are reinforced. Second, the day school system encourages endogamous marriage. Romance is much more likely to blossom when teens are in the same social circles, circles which are created through their schoolmates. Finally, the day school system places an equal emphasis on Jewish and secular learning. The importance of Jewish education is reinforced by a parental desire to see their children succeed both academically and spiritually.

It is almost always the mothers who make the trek to Baltimore each day, which I suspect is in large part due to their husband's obligations to be at the morning *minyan* at the temple. The mothers have organized themselves into a carpool, with the few homemakers taking on a larger percentage of the driving. Clearly the time spent at school reinforces the children's Orthodox identity, but the importance of the commute should not be overlooked. It is during this time that the children are made acutely aware that they are not like other children in Lancaster. Their lives are also not like the other students in their day school. Despite these differences, the importance of their family's commitment to Orthodoxy is underscored as they drive three hours each day to and from Baltimore.

For those families that choose not to, or cannot afford to, enroll their children in Baltimore's day school, their children can receive additional Jewish education through Degel Israel's Hebrew School. Unlike local Reform and Conservative programs which meet once a week, Degel Israel's program meets twice weekly and more often if the student is preparing for a bar/bat mitzvah. These classes, save for private bar/bat mitzvah study with the Rabbi, are entirely taught by women. The synagogue's educational plan and curriculum is overseen by the Rebbetzin. She, along with her daughters and occasionally other women, teach all of the classes. Women are responsible for the Jewish education of Degel Israel's children both in the home and in the synagogue.

In addition to volunteering as Hebrew School teachers, the synagogue's female membership volunteers in countless other ways. The women are involved both in the synagogue and the community. At Degel Israel, they prepare dinner each night for the students at the Lancaster Yeshiva Center, teach Hebrew School twice a week, prepare a weekly *Kiddush*, arrange all special community meals, take part in fundraising efforts, work to landscape and garden the grounds, visit the sick and elderly, learn Torah with other women, and the list goes on. Their volunteerism does not stop within the synagogue walls. They also send frequent care packages to troops overseas, work as greeters and volunteer receptionists at local hospitals, provide childcare, work with Meals-on-Wheels, speak to local churches and church groups about religious diversity—all of this alongside of their family, career, religious and social commitments.

After considering their long list of volunteerism, remember how small the congregation is. It is astounding how much these women accomplish each day. They are the face of the Lancaster Orthodox community and, although they are too humble to admit it, they are also the heart. Without their tireless efforts, careful preparation, and intense commitment to Orthodoxy, the community would fall apart. They feed, protect, nurture and educate their families, all the while working and volunteering. It is through the efforts of the women of Degel Israel that many of the hurdles of living in a small community are overcome. This is not to negate the struggles of local male Orthodoxy, but it is the labors of the women that combat the pressures to assimilate. Through their dedication, the women enable the synagogue to collectively thrive.

Until the local Orthodox population grows, the work of these women is never done. It is a long and difficult road ahead of them, as they fight to keep their community alive. However, much like they embark on their daily commute to Baltimore to bring their children to school, they steer their families and community down the road—always looking forward.

NOTES

1. Ira M. Sheskin, *Geographical Differences Among American* Jews (New York: National Jewish Population Survey, 2004), 5.

2. Sheskin, *Geographical Differences*, 7.

3. Sheskin, *Geographical Differences*, 5.

4. Sheskin, *Geographical Differences*, 7.

5. Sheskin, *Geographical Differences*, 9. 28 percent of the Jewish population over the age of 65 lives in the South.

6. Sheskin, *Geographical Differences*, 10.

7. Sheskin, *Geographical Differences*, 9–11.

8. Sheskin, *Geographical Differences*, 15.

9. Sheskin, *Geographical Differences*, 20.

10. The Jewish Federations of North America, "National Jewish Population Survey: Orthodox Jews, 2001, http://www.jewishfederations.org/local_includes/downloads/4983.pdf (accessed June 22, 2011), 15.

11. Sheskin, *Geographical Differences*, 16–17, 20–21.

12. The Jewish Federations of North America, "National Jewish Population Survey," 19.

13. The Jewish Federations of North America, "National Jewish Population Survey," 5.

14. The Jewish Federations of North America, "National Jewish Population Survey," 8.

15. The Jewish Federations of North America, "National Jewish Population Survey," 7.

16. The Jewish Federations of North America, "National Jewish Population Survey," 10.

17. The Jewish Federations of North America, "National Jewish Population Survey," 9.

18. The Jewish Federations of North America, "National Jewish Population Survey," 10.

19. The Jewish Federations of North America, "National Jewish Population Survey," 11.

20. The Jewish Federations of North America, "National Jewish Population Survey," 12.

21. National Vital Statistics Report, "Births," 2011, http://www.cdc.gov/nchs/data/nvsr/nvsr59/nvsr59_03.pdf (accessed July 19, 2011).

22. Jack Wertheimer, "Low Fertility and High Intermarriage are Pushing American Jewry Toward Extinction," 2011 http://www.aish.com/jw/s/48899452.html (accessed July 19, 2011).

23. The Jewish Federations of North America, "National Jewish Population Survey," 13.

24. The Jewish Federations of North America, "National Jewish Population Survey," 21.

25. The Jewish Federations of North America, "National Jewish Population Survey," 17.

26. See David Brener, *The Jews of Lancaster, Pennsylvania: A Story with Two beginnings* (Lancaster: PA: Congregation Shaarai Shomayim, 1979).

27. US Census, "Lancaster County, Pennsylvania," 2011b, http://www.quickfacts.census.gov/qfd/states/41/42071/html (accessed January 6, 2011).

28. US Census, "Lancaster (city), Pennsylvania," 2011a, http://quickfacts.census.gov/qfd/states/41/4241216.html (accessed January 6, 2011).

29. Association of Religion Data Archives, "Lancaster County, Pennsylvania," 2010a, http://www.thearda.com/mapsReports/reports/counties/42071_2000.asp (accessed December 28, 2010).

30. Association of Religion Data Archives, "The United States, General," 2010b, http://www.thearda.com/internationalData/countries/Country_234_1.asp (accessed December 28, 2010).

31. Association of Religion Data Archives, "The United States, General."

32. Ira Sheskin and Arnold Dashefsky, *Jewish Population in the United States, 2010* (Storrs, CT: Jewish Data Bank and the Jewish Federations of North America, 2010), 20.

33. Sheskin and Sashefsky, *Jewish Population*, 43.

34. Sheskin and Sashefsky, *Jewish Population*, 66.

35. Ira Sheskin, "Recent Trends in Jewish Demographics and Their Impact on the Jewish Media," 2011, http://www.jewishdatabank.org/Reports/RecentTrends_Sheskin_2011/pdf (accessed June 20, 2011).

36. Etan Diamond, *And I Will Dwell in Their Midst: Orthodox Jews in Suburbia*, (Chapel Hill: University of North Carolina Press, 2000), 5.

37. Diamond, *And I Will Dwell in Their Midst*, 5; see Marshall Sklare, *Jewish Identity on the Suburban Frontier: A Study of Group Survival in the Open Society* (Chicago: University of Chicago Press, 1967); Lee Shai Weissbach, *Jewish Life in Small-Town America: A History* (New Haven: Yale University Press, 2005).

38. United Jewish Communities, "Jews in Small Communities," 2011, http://www.jewishfederations.org/local_includes/downloads/5542.pdf (accessed June 23, 2011), 3.

39. United Jewish Communities, "Jews in Small Communities," 6–7.

40. United Jewish Communities, "Jews in Small Communities," 8, 28.

41. United Jewish Communities, "Jews in Small Communities," 9–10.

42. United Jewish Communities, "Jews in Small Communities," 29.

43. United Jewish Communities, "Jews in Small Communities," 31.

44. United Jewish Communities, "Jews in Small Communities," 13–14.

45. United Jewish Communities, "Jews in Small Communities," 15.

46. United Jewish Communities, "Jews in Small Communities," 16.

47. United Jewish Communities, "Jews in Small Communities," 25–26.

48. United Jewish Communities, "Jews in Small Communities," 17, 20.

49. Solomon Poll, *The Hasidic Community of Williamsburg: A Study in the Sociology of Religion* (New York: Free Press, 1962), 59–69. Poll identifies dress as marking six Hasidic social classes. Still, within these classes, there is a homogeneity and sense of collective identification.

50. As will be seen in later chapters, particularly chapter five, not all of the members' children will continue to identify as Orthodox Jews.

51. The correct movie quote is actually, "If you build it, he will come." However, popular repetition of this line has over time rendered it, "If you build it, they will come."

52. Shaya Sackett, "The Lancaster Yeshiva Center," 2011, http://www.lancasteryeshiva.com (accessed June 25, 2011).

53. An example of the tension between Orthodoxy and urban communities is the Crown Heights Riot. This three day riot began on August 19, 1991, when an African American child was hit and killed by a car driven by a Hasidic man. The event brought racial tensions to the surface and property was destroyed, individuals injured, and homes and businesses were burglarized. Ultimately the community would come together and work toward teaching others about tolerance through the Crown Heights Coalition and the Crown Heights Mediation Center.

54. See Jewish Orthodox Feminist Alliance, "Bat Mitzvah," 2011a, http://www.jofa.org/social.php/life/batmiztvah (accessed June 28, 2011); Ora Wiskind Elper, *Traditions and Celebrations of the Bat Mitzvah* (New York: Urim, 2003).

55. There was one particularly scandalous bat mitzvah where one young woman chanted Torah in a situation where men were not expecting to hear her voice. It is an event that is still frequently discussed.

56. During the summer of 2011 the kosher food stand at Dutch Wonderland Amusement Park in Lancaster, Pennsylvania, announced that it would begin carrying pizza. Although not open year round, there is now opportunity to purchase kosher pizza locally during the summer months. However, priced at almost $22.00 per plain pizza, many women still prefer the cheaper method of purchasing pizza in Baltimore and freezing it for future use.

57. It is true that there are some staples that are available at the local grocery stores—vegetables and certain packaged goods, for example. However, as several of the women have pointed out numerous times, "You can't live on Oreos alone!" Oreos, incidentally, had their kosher certification reinstated during the writing of this manuscript, much to the joy of several members of the Lancaster community.

Chapter Four

Wearing Many Hats

The Hair Covering Practices of the Orthodox Jewish Women at Degel Israel Synagogue

Our meeting had just concluded, and Vicki and I parted ways. Nearly four hours had passed in a local coffee shop as we got to know one another and chatted about hair covering. Deciding to get one last refill before I drove home, I approached the counter alone. As I waited for my coffee, another customer rested her hand on my arm. "It's such a great thing that you are supporting your friend as she goes through this difficult time. I'm sure it means a lot to her," she nodded reassuringly. The blank look on my face elicited an attempt at clarification. "When I had my cancer, it was friends like you that kept me going," she explained. I smiled, responding, "She doesn't have cancer. She's an Orthodox Jew."

The case of mistaken identity is not unusual for Orthodox women. Although hair covering is a concrete expression of observance that serves to differentiate levels of religiosity and group allegiance to those within Orthodoxy, it is more often than not a misunderstood or misassigned marker for society at large. This is especially true for the Orthodox women in Lancaster, Pennsylvania. Those who cover their hair are often mistaken for Mennonites or questioned about hair loss. In a locale where most assume there are few, if any, Jews, many are surprised to discover a small religiously observant Orthodox community tucked away in the heart of Amish country. Area residents are aware with the head coverings worn by the sizable local Amish and Mennonite population; yet, they are generally unfamiliar with the hair covering practices of Orthodox Jewish women. Stemming from *minhag*, Orthodox women cover their hair after marriage as a *siman nisuin* (Hebrew for sign of marriage). Although much of contemporary Jewry has abandoned this practice, it still exhibits a foothold within Orthodoxy. However, removed from larger urban settings where communities are familiar with their Orthodox neighbors, the Jewish women of Degel Israel Synagogue often find themselves misunderstood. Likewise, their role has gone largely unrecognized by the academy. There have been few comprehensive studies completed of Orthodox women living outside of urban and suburban areas. These women exist on the periphery of both their local community and academic scholarship.

AMERICAN WIG CULTURE

This chapter begins by offering an introduction to American wig culture. Following this overview, I offer an introduction to the women interviewed to help contextualize their hair covering choices. In addition to consideration of the women's explanations of their personal motivations, this contextualized approach also considers motivations that may exist outside of their awareness. This serves as the basis of my analysis, which argues that the diversity of hair covering practices helps to create boundaries that enable the women, through self-identification, to negotiate the tensions of living in a small religious community.

Wigs—their look, style, function, and popularity—have evolved and changed over time. We will begin by first considering the historic evolution of the wig, taking into account both its ancient roots and contemporary application. We will then discuss contemporary American wig culture, concentrating on the three main groups of wig wearers: African American women, women with health issues, and Orthodox women.

Since ancient times there has been a desire to alter the appearance using wigs. Hairpieces were worn by both sexes, although the style varied based on age, gender, and social status. The appeal of wigs was largely influenced by health reasons or expressions of class. Ancient Egyptians, for example, shaved their heads to avoid lice. Likewise, wealthy individuals would wear wigs made of hair from slaves or the deceased. Those from lower socioeconomic classes wore wigs made of grass or purchased a partial wig to which they could later add additional hair extensions. [1]

The popularity of wigs continued during the Roman Empire. Wigs were popular across class lines, although their quality and style served as a clear indication of class. It was during the Roman period that the idea of wigs marking professions emerged. Prostitutes, for example, were required to either bleach their hair or wear blonde wigs. Dark hair indicated refinement and membership in the upper class. [2]

Wig wearing encountered its first major setback during the Middle Ages. The Catholic Church frowned upon hairpieces, citing them as ostentatious and frivolous, and encouraged short natural hairstyles. King Henry IV even went so far as to ban wigs. Despite these tensions, long hair was still considered beautiful, and men and women were willing to go to great lengths in order to achieve a luxurious head of hair. By the mid-1500s clergy became more accepting of hairpieces. With this change, partial hairpieces which were incorporated into elaborate hairstyles crept their way into the daily hair styles of most middle- and upper-class Europeans. The popularity of wigs continued to grow through the 1600s, especially when others emulated the coiffure of noted individuals like Queen Elizabeth I, Mary Queen of Scots, King Louis XIII, and King Charles II.[3]

Wig culture drastically changed in the late 1700s and 1800s. The affordability of wigs increased, allowing individuals of all socioeconomic classes the ability to purchase hairpieces. Human hair wigs were preferred by the upper classes, but horse, goat, or yak hair was also used to create more affordable wig alternatives.[4] Much like hats indicate cultural shifts—for example, becoming larger and more ornate for wealthy theater goers when theater became more affordable for the masses—wigs also signify cultural change. Fearful of the blurring of class distinctions, the elite used wigs as status symbols, not only purchasing wigs made of high quality hair, but also styling and adorning them in ornate and grandiose ways. The wealthy wore wigs that could rise several feet above their heads. As Victoria Sherrow describes it, "[these] wigs were further adorned with gemstones, feathers, flowers, fruits, vegetables, garlands, and other trimmings. Some women created entire scenes on their heads—rooms full of miniature furniture, arrangements of small children's toys or musical instruments, gardens, birdcages with real birds inside, and detailed model ships."[5]

Wig culture in early America was quite similar to the European experience. Early Puritans frowned upon wigs, believing that they blurred the distinction between genders. Despite this warning, many early settlers still wore hairpieces. Like Europe, wigs served as an American status symbol. Whether it was the size, quality, and style of the wig or the ability to purchase multiple hairpieces (as was the case with Southern plantation owners who bought wigs for their housekeepers, butlers, or other slaves who worked in the home), hairpieces made a strong statement of social class.[6]

Americans gradually lost interest in wigs. After the Revolutionary War, Americans were increasingly interested in abolishing class distinctions and moving away from their dependence on Europe. One of the ways in which they accomplished this was in the abandonment of wig culture and in the development of a new American fashion sense. Despite this change, smaller hairpieces were still used by Victorian women to enhance their elaborate hairstyles;[7] however, as hairstyles simplified and the focus of interest shifted to hats, Americans increasingly ignored wigs.

American wig consciousness was rattled during the 1960s with the advent of the popular bouffant hairstyle. Wigs and hairpieces reemerged as methods to add increased length or height to hair—especially to create styles like the bouffant or the beehive.[8] However, when long flowing locks came into style during the 1970s, wigs once again decreased in popularity. The contemporary American wig industry now focuses on three primary groups of clientele: African American women, women with health issues, and Orthodox Jewish women.

Many African American women have a complicated relationship with their hair. American society teaches that a beautiful woman has long, flowing, straight locks. Even when curly hair is in vogue, the length and texture of the hair's curl still defines its appeal. In other words, "white hair" defines what is beautiful. Not all African American women are able to grow their hair beyond a certain length. If they do grow their hair, many engage in a constant battle to wrangle it into an unnatural state. Those women who embrace natural hair are faced with harsh societal reactions. They are told that their hair is "nappy" or "unkempt." They must face stereotypes that African American women with natural hair are "likely to be man-haters, feminists, or lesbians." As Althea Prince sums up the tension of natural versus straightened hair, "These are harsh stereotypes to live with, especially if you are young, vulnerable about your self-image, and trying to find love."[9]

African American women embraced the flapper hairstyles of the 1920s, enjoying the stylistic freedom that the short-bob haircuts afforded them. However, as hairstyles lengthened in the 1930s, African American women began mail ordering hairpieces and wigs to lengthen their hair or to help create and maintain straight styles.[10] The styles of the World War II era, characterized for African American women by the short haircuts of Lena Horne and Dorothy Dandridge, posed another problem. Although these hairstyles were short, they were also essentially straight. The use of "falsies," small hairpieces also known as "switches," flourished as African American women used them to achieve the popular short tapered hairstyles.[11]

Although big hair enjoyed a certain degree of popularity during the 1960s and 1970s,[12] the use of hair straightening, weaves, falls, and hairpieces has endured as part of African American female hair styling. Now a billion dollar industry, African American hair supplies have had an enormous impact on American hair culture. Hair weaves, pioneered by African American women, are now popular with women of all races and the stigma attached to using false hair has decreased. Popular celebrities, including Oprah Winfrey, Tyra Banks, Raven-Symoné, and Kim Kardashian, have admitted to using hair extensions, which has helped to change American views on wiggery.

Still, when Americans speak of wigs, they most commonly think of cancer patients. In fact, wigs and hair coverings are frequently marketed toward women with hair loss, particularly those who have lost their hair due to medical reasons. Sometimes medical treatment causes hair loss as is the case in cancer patients. Other instances of baldness or balding stem from genetic causes like alopecia.

Regardless of the reason for hair loss, an entire industry has developed around the covering of hair loss, particularly female baldness. Whether they use hats, turbans, head scarves, or wigs, women experiencing hair loss have a wide variety of choices at their disposal. Entire support groups have developed, both public and online, for women to discuss the impact that hair loss has had on their lives. Likewise, charitable organizations have formed to help offset the expense of purchasing a wig. The most recognizable group is the popular *Locks of Love*, an organization that collects donated human hair to create wigs for children experiencing hair loss. Other organizations, like *Pantene Beautiful Lengths*, collect and donate hair to create wigs for women who have lost their hair due to cancer treatment. The American Cancer Society also maintains "wig banks," which help match individuals with hair pieces, styling services, or wig cleaning.

The final group actively participating in the American wig industry is Orthodox Jewish women. Although their numbers are significantly less than the aforementioned groups, they still profoundly influence American wiggery. They do not see their wigs as temporary investments, as cancer patients might, nor are they interested in partial hairpieces, as are many African American women. Instead, Orthodox women consider their *sheitels* (wigs) an investment, often purchasing several high-end human hair wigs that they maintain concurrently.

Orthodox Jewish women began using wigs to cover their hair during the sixteenth century. As wigs became secularly popular for both sexes, Jewish women embraced wigs as a hair covering method that did not force them to define themselves publicly as "other."[13] Rabbinic authorities struggled to determine whether or not a wig constituted a proper hair covering. Some, like sixteenth century Rabbi Katzenellenbogen, maintained that wigs were immodest and not sufficient hair covering. For Katzenellenbogen, although the letter of the law was upheld, wigs violated the spirit of the law. In this view, although the woman's hair is technically covered, the fact that a wig appears as hair to the eyes of observers, especially male viewers, means that a woman actually appears uncovered.[14] Other authorities, like Rabbi Moshe Isserles, asserted that wigs met the *halakhic* requirements of hair covering.[15] In this view, the importance is in the daily act of covering the hair. In doing so, the literal parameters of *halakha* are met.

This centuries-long debate has still not been resolved. It is commonly accepted that most modern *Ashkenazic* women embrace the wig as a valid means of hair covering, while most *Sephardic* Jews reject wigs.[16] However, this division is not always accurate. Orthodox women make many choices about their bodies and self-presentation. Their hair covering choices have exhibited greater influence over the debate than rabbinic authority. As Leila Bronner notes, "Despite their lack of formal *halakhic* influence, [Orthodox women] made a statement through their continued wearing of the wig in the face of rabbinic opposition."[17] Indeed, it is their lived practice and embodiment of hair covering that has determined its cultural acceptability. As will be demonstrated by the women profiled in this chapter, great thought goes into the decision of whether or not to wear a *sheitel*. This decision is influenced by individual preference as well as certain social contexts.

HAIR COVERING PRACTICES AT DEGEL ISRAEL SYNAGOGUE

Six women are profiled in this study of the women who cover their hair at Degel Israel: Chaya, Debbie, Haddasah, Kathy, Naomi, and Vicki. Eight female Degel Israel members currently engage in full time hair covering practices. Two were unable to participate in this study. One, a Modern Orthodox woman had scheduling conflicts and the other, a member of the Chabad Lubavitch Hasidim, did not respond to inquiries. In addition to these eight women, there are at least three women who cover their hair only at religious services.

I gathered information on these six women during interviews I conducted between October and December, 2010. The women were asked a set list of thirty questions in order to establish a basis for comparison, but they were also encouraged to share personal anecdotes and opinions. Interviews generally lasted about an hour and a half, with the longest running into its fourth hour. Four women chose to meet in their homes, while two elected to meet in a local coffee shop.

The women range in age from 49 to 58. All married, they each have between one and five children. Although only Chaya's mother covers her hair, all of their married daughters and daughters-in-law cover their hair. All of the women are high school graduates; Chaya and Vicki attended college, and Kathy and Debbie hold graduate degrees. With the exception of Naomi, all of the women are employed outside of the home. Their professions include owning and operating a well-known local business, writing a newspaper column, working as a prominent attorney, serving as president of a telecommunications business, and overseeing Jewish educational programming.

Although all of the women are affiliated with Orthodoxy, they classify themselves differently. Chaya prefers the term "Observant" to Orthodox because of the variety of ways that the word can be interpreted. Likewise, Debbie prefers to be called "Torah-observant." Kathy and Naomi self-identify solely as "Orthodox;" Vicki considers herself "Modern Orthodox," and

Haddasah specifies that she is a member of the Belz Hasidim. All six women keep kosher kitchens and are *shomer shabbos*.

Not all of the women were raised in observant families. Only Chaya and Haddasah were raised within an Orthodox family. Vicki and Debbie were both raised in Conservative families and consider themselves *ba'alot teshuva* (Jews who recommit themselves to Judaism and begin to live a religiously observant lifestyle). Naomi has a hard time classifying her past. Although she was raised in a family where she wore pants, her upbringing was somewhat observant. From her description, her family seems to fall somewhere between the hybrid label of "Conservadox" and Modern Orthodox. Kathy, raised a United Methodist, had a Conservative conversion when she was married. Later, as she and her husband became more observant, she underwent a second Orthodox conversion. Similarly, not all of the women began covering their hair immediately after they married. Only Chaya and Haddasah, not coincidentally the only two raised Orthodox, covered immediately after marriage. Kathy, Vicki, Debbie, and Naomi would come to cover as they became more religiously observant.

The women use a variety of methods to cover their hair. Unlike other communities where hair covering choices are more standardized, the women at Degel Israel have the autonomy to choose which type of hair covering best suits them and meets their needs. Chaya wears a *sheitel* (wig) outside of the synagogue. On the Sabbath or when teaching at the Hebrew school, she wears a hat or a snood (a close-fitting hood that encases the hair in a small sack). She does this to ensure that it is clear that her hair is covered, as a good *sheitel* can go undetected. Although Vicki, Kathy, Haddasah, and Naomi own *sheitels*, they rarely wear them, generally saving them only for weddings or other special events. Naomi favors pre-tied *tichels* (scarves) and wears them almost exclusively. Vicki, on the other hand, wears a variety of *tichels*, hats, and snoods. Kathy is known as "the hat lady" by her colleagues. She has a large collection of hats, ranging from understated to eye catching. She has made hats her fashion trademark, which she believes helps to keep others focused on her professional role rather than her religious observance. Haddasah greatly dislikes her *sheitel* and rarely wears it, unless she feels that a social situation necessitates it. She wears snoods and pre-tied *tichels*, but sadly laments that she does not live in a community where *shpitzels* (a head covering worn by some Hasidic women that has a braid of hair across the front and is covered by a *tichel*) are the norm. Debbie is the only woman who never wears a *sheitel*. She feels strongly that they defeat the purpose of hair covering. She ties her own *tichels* and even had a custom-made *tichel* created to match the dress she recently wore to her son's wedding.

Of the six women interviewed, only Naomi dyes and professionally styles her hair. Kathy will occasionally have a professional haircut, but also trims her own hair. Vicki, Debbie, and Chaya all cut their own hair and do not color it. It is only in recent years that Haddasah has allowed her hair to grow out. Previously, like some other Hasidic women, she had kept her head shaved, but now she trims the ends as needed.

Another significant variation is whether or not the women keep their hair covered at all times. Both Chaya and Haddasah cover their hair constantly, even when sleeping.[18] Vicki and Debbie cover their hair at all times while awake, but do not cover their hair when asleep. Kathy and Naomi both keep their hair covered when outside of the house or when guests are visiting. However, when in the home and in the presence of immediate family or select close female friends, they do not always keep their hair covered.

The final striking difference between the women is their attendance at religious services. Although all of the women are *shomer shabbos*, only Chaya and Naomi attend most all of the Saturday morning services at Degel Israel. Debbie is equally as active, but almost always chooses to attend services at the larger Orthodox synagogue in Harrisburg, Pennsylvania. Kathy attends about half of Sabbath services; however, Vicki and Haddasah never attend services or other events at Degel Israel. For many years both Haddasah and Vicki participated in Saturday morning services, but after some social tensions arose between their families and the Rabbi's family, only their husbands continue to attend services.

HAIR AND *YIDDISHKEIT*

The women of Degel Israel exist as a quadruple minority. That is to say, as Jews they already are within an American minority group. Within Judaism, Orthodoxy is the minority, and within their local secular community, they are the extreme minority. In addition, they represent the few among Degel Israel who chose to cover their hair. They are geographically situated in an area unfamiliar with Judaism, especially Orthodoxy. Their beliefs and lifestyle are both unusual and foreign to their neighbors. Even those within their community do not always understand and support their religious choices. Haddasah describes her experience, saying, "Most of the people in this community don't think like me at all. I have loads of friends online, other *Hasidische* women. I need that. I didn't think I was going to need it [when I moved to Lancaster], but I do."[19] Vicki quips, "I mean, really, a Jewish woman's worst enemy is, well, another Jewish woman. I honestly feel that way. If you don't go along with the crowd, they try to make you an outcast. That's sometimes what I feel, but it's mostly in small communities. If we were in a larger community, certain people wouldn't even be here. They would have moved out [of Degel Israel] a long time ago. They wouldn't have been tolerated."

If the same group of women were to be located in an area with a higher Orthodox population, in addition to subdividing into separate religious communities, they also would find themselves subject to greater social pressures to conform. Rather than having social control imposed upon them by their neighbors and religious community, the women at Degel Israel self-elect to uphold religious laws. Their Christian neighbors would not know the difference if they drove on the Sabbath or if they did not cover their hair. The Lancaster Orthodox community would continue to accept them regardless of their choices. Why then do these women embrace hair covering? I contend that there are three primary motivations: externalization of their religious commitment, marking of their level of observance, and their children.

With the exception of Haddasah and Chaya, the other women have all had a turning point in their religious lives where they recommitted themselves to Judaism. Debra Renee Kaufman's analysis in *Rachel's Daughters: Newly Orthodox Jewish Women* is helpful when considering the motivations of the women of Degel Israel. Kaufman only briefly addresses hair and hair covering in her work, but she clearly considers hair an expressive marker of religious devotion.[20] In the case of newly Orthodox women, hair functions as a demonstrable sign of Orthodox conversion to both the wearer and the viewer. This is especially true because of its prominent place on the head, demonstrating both an individual choice and an acceptance of a group established collective appearance.

Both the women in Kaufman's case study and the women at Degel Israel use their hair as an expression of their *Yiddishkeit* (Jewishness). They move away from the secular world in which they were raised and use their hair to mark themselves as newly and decidedly Orthodox. Although the women in Kaufman's study frequently stated their distaste and mistrust for what they perceived as a hypersexualized society, the women of Degel Israel rarely speak of the secular world in terms of sex. Rather, they focus on the emptiness that they felt before they increased their level of observance. Indeed, it is through this spiritual seeking of truth that they have turned to Orthodoxy. Through the reappropriation of their hair from fashion to sacred, they mark themselves as part of a religious community that is decidedly different from the secular culture they knew earlier. It is their way of distinguishing themselves from their neighbors, families, and previous lifestyle, as well as realigning themselves with their new community.

In their Lancaster County context, this idea of living as religiously other is familiar to their secular neighbors. The women may not theologically agree with the local Amish and Mennonite residents. Anabaptists comprise almost 12 percent of the local population[21] but they express a certain degree of empathy and understanding about countercultural lifestyle choices. Haddasah explains, "I'm always being asked what I am . . . I have a lot of Amish friends. They kind of understand the whole thing. But they ask me, "Do you cover your hair for the same reason that we are [sic]?" Maybe not exactly, but I'm not going to get into a whole big thing about it. I just say, "Yes, that's it." You know, for religious reasons." Debbie also finds the area to be fairly tolerant of religious clothing choices because of the local Anabaptist population. She recounts, "When my son was younger, I never had a problem letting him go into the movie theater bathroom or anything with his *yarmulke*. 'Cause most people in Lancaster wouldn't know a *yarmulke* from a hat. There's [sic] so many people walking around here with different stuff on their heads, no one notices anymore."

In their move towards Orthodoxy, these women took on several other important Jewish rituals. They uphold the laws of *niddah* (sexual purity), keep kosher homes, and are *shomer shabbos*. None of these, however, is easily demonstrable publicly. Whether it is for their extended families, their local community, or even themselves, hair covering serves as an external marker of their observance of these other rituals. This externalization also helps to negotiate and establish distinct gender roles, which they believe the secular world to have blurred. Their hair covering indicates observance within the Orthodox community and, perhaps even more importantly in the Lancaster context, marks them as Jewish women to their secular neighbors. Just as their husbands and sons wear *kippot* (skullcaps) and *tzitzit* (knotted ritual fringes), these women use hair covering as a public performance of belief. They are not only privately Jews in the home, but also publicly Jews on the street.

Hair covering can easily be forgone in such a small and diverse community. Indeed, when initial inquiries were made concerning which women covered outside of Sabbath services, community members struggled to reach a consensus. Living in relative isolation from one another, Degel Israel members do not always have full social knowledge of their religious community. The social pressure that one might experience in a more homogenous community does not exert the same form of control. They must then choose to self-regulate their hair covering practices. For the most part, other synagogue members would have no way of knowing if these women chose to forgo their head coverings during the work week, which is a much different experience than Orthodox women who live in predominantly Jewish neighborhoods.

Several of the women interviewed mentioned Azriela Jaffe's book, *What Do You Mean, You Can't Eat in My Home?: A Guide to How Newly Observant Jews and Their Less Observant Relatives Can Still Get Along.* [22] Jaffe, a former Lancaster resident, is a prominent writer, professional speaker, and Jewish educator. Writing extensively on Jewish topics, she specializes in the role of Orthodox women in the family, especially in terms of negotiating traditionalism with modernity. Several of the Lancaster women pointed to Jaffe as an example of the importance of hair covering. Although Jaffe had been a popular hostess in the Lancaster community, the women recount that after relocating to New Jersey, members of her new synagogue were not receptive to her invitations. Finally, after several months, she directly questioned another synagogue member. She was told that it was because of her hair covering choices that others chose not to dine in her home. They were unsure if she kept an adequately kosher kitchen because of her uncovered hair.[23]

This anecdote clearly expresses the anxieties of the women of Degel Israel. Even those who adhere to the most meticulous of private observances could be mistaken for unobservant if they failed to cover their hair. When recommitting themselves to Judaism, all four women identified their first step as keeping a kosher kitchen—including the prohibition of nonkosher foods, maintaining separate utensils, plates, and cookware for dairy and meat, the *kashering* (rendering something kosher) of sinks, glassware, and dishwashers, and the removal of all nonkosher items. As they increased their level of observance, they struggled with the idea of hair covering. As Debbie describes it, "It's usually the last thing people do [when they become observant]. It's the most noticeable for people to question you about. You're doing something that everyone sees. Keeping a kosher home, no one has to see." Raised in synagogues where hair covering was not normative and living in a community where most Orthodox Jewish women did not cover required the newly religious women of Degel Israel to exhibit a significant commitment to Orthodox Judaism. Beginning to publicly cover their hair othered them from their secular life and was, in all cases, the final step in the recommitment process.

The women at Degel Israel, in line with much of contemporary Orthodoxy, distinguish between "FFB" and "BT"—shorthand for "*frum* from birth," which refers to those who were raised Orthodox and *ba'alot teshuva*, women who have recommitted themselves to Judaism. Using hair covering as a means of distinguishing themselves as religiously observant is not only important to those who have increased their religious observance over time. Haddasah and Chaya, the only two who are considered FFB, use hair covering as a marker of their own longstanding commitment to the religious lifestyle. Chaya describes the importance she sees of covering her hair saying, "You feel like you are observing another commandment, even though it is a more implicit than explicit commandment. You feel like, you know, it is another thing you are doing to be observant. And also, you feel like this gives me the status that I know that I cover my hair."

None of the women interviewed is a native of Lancaster County. Except for Naomi, all of the women who identify as BT had relocated to the area prior to recommitting themselves to Judaism.[24] Haddasah and Chaya, on the other hand, already covered their hair when they moved to Lancaster. Entering a community where there was such a vast diversity within Orthodoxy, hair covering was the outwardly expressive way that the two were able to mark themselves as religiously observant. For both women, it was unthinkable that they would cease to cover their hair after relocating. They were both fully committed to the practice, as it was an integral part of their self-identity as an Orthodox Jewish woman.[25] Haddasah reminisces, "Before [in Brooklyn], there were women who covered their hair everywhere. Very *frum*. Very *tznius* (modest). But now, you know, I'm more alone. By myself."[26]

Several women articulated the difficulty of moving to a small community. Naomi muses, "From going to a big city to going to this, well it's a change. Yes, a big change from Baltimore. Usually it's the other way around. You move from here to the city." Haddasah agrees, noting, "This is a challenge sometimes. It is really hard. There are a lot more politics involved here. There are much more than there are in Brooklyn, 'cause everybody is, well, there are just so few [Orthodox] here." Unlike the others, Chaya, Naomi and Haddasah know what it was like to live in a larger Orthodox community. Although all of the women expressed the great difficulty experienced when living in an area with such a small Orthodox population, these three, in particular, mused over how much easier it is to live in an Orthodox neighborhood.[27] Haddasah explained, "It's everything. The food, the people, neighborhood, community. Now the only other modestly dressed women I see are Mennonites."

Chaya and Haddasah's decision to continue to cover their hair, even when the community around them does not, seems to indicate a desire to maintain a connection to the communities that they left. Particularly in the case of Haddasah, who strongly identifies herself as a member of the Belz Hasidim of which only she and her husband are members in Lancaster County—her hair covering choices indicate her continued self-identification with the larger Belz community. Although Belz Hasidim can be found throughout the world, they are particularly concentrated in Israel and Brooklyn, New York (mostly the Borough Park section). After near obliteration during the Holocaust, they have rebounded to become the one of the largest Hasidic groups in Borough Park. As Samuel Heilman describes the group, Belz Hasidim are "associated with extreme counteracculturationist views, rejecting all compromises with secularity."[28] After relocating to Lancaster for employment, Haddasah and her husband are living in a cultural diaspora, separated from the rest of their religious community. Hair covering is one way that Haddasah can forge a connection between the group that they desire to be a part of and their reality.

For all of the women, their choice to cover their hair is perhaps most important in terms of the greater, rather than the local, Orthodox community. All six women are mothers and consider their hair covering to have a crucial impact on their children. They indicate this occurring on two levels. First, the women consider their choice to cover their hair a critical demonstration to their children of the importance of religious observance. As Chaya explains, "Mothers mold their kids. Moms make a Jewish home Jewish, you know, showing their kids what's important. When she covers her hair, she shows them that, well, she's not afraid to be a Jew when she's not in *shul* (synagogue) or at home. You know, like saying to her kids that she's a Jew 24/7." In other words, these women believe that through their choice to cover, their children will realize the significance of living an Orthodox lifestyle. Although they all indicate that this is the case for both boys and girls. The women seem particularly concerned with their daughters' future spirituality and practice. Collectively, the women, as a result of their educational choices for their children and their own role modeling, have attempted to instill in their children the importance and benefits of religious observance.

The second level that the women see as an impact on their children is in the matchmaking process. As they look for *shidduchim* (matches) for their children, they are very aware of the role that their hair covering plays in the process. Some will use a *shadchan* (professional Orthodox matchmaker), in this case from Baltimore, who will question whether or not potential mates' mothers cover their hair, as well as whether or not the unmarried female intends to cover her hair after marriage. It serves as a strong indicator of the level of religious observance adhered to by the individuals and their families. Lack of hair covering could potentially have a detrimental impact on the matchmaking process. As Kathy explains, "If it were just me, I might not ever wear a *sheitel* [instead of a hat]. This may sound crass, but I do it for the sake of my children, for their *shidduchim*."

The women of Degel Israel are acutely aware of the importance of their hair covering choices in the matchmaking process. Unlike other communities where families are familiar with each other and live locally, their children are forced to seek *shidduchim* outside of the Lancaster community. There simply are not enough young Orthodox singles at Degel Israel, nor are they all seeking the same level of observance in potential mates. With prospective families that are unfamiliar with them, both the interested youth and their parents have to establish themselves in the eyes of potential partners. Hair covering, in this regard, functions as a form of matchmaking currency. Chaya explains, "You cover your hair—that means you have a certain level of observancy. It's a barometer. Fair or not fair, it's a barometer." It is an evaluative tool that individuals and families use to assess the level of religious observance of their possible *shidduchim*.

With no local Orthodox Jewish day schools in the area and inability to relocate as a result of their employment, Kathy, Chaya, Debbie, and Naomi all chose to send their children to Orthodox schools in Baltimore, requiring a daily commute of over an hour each way. This choice helped to ensure that their children would build up a social network in Baltimore, which has a sizable Orthodox Jewish population. Of these women, only Debbie and Chaya have married children; their matches were all made through their Baltimore connections. Both feel that their choice to cover their hair impacted their children's *shidduchim*. Chaya elaborates, "In fact, [my daughters] looked for a spouse who would want his wife to cover her hair, because that shows a level of commitment, and they want someone who is at that same level of commitment that they are. Just makes it so much easier. If you hook up with a guy who it doesn't matter [to], that already shows that you aren't on the same wavelength. So, the more you have in common, the better it is. You know, you start on an even plateau as you embark on marriage."

Kathy feels additional pressure to cover her hair in order to enhance her children's matchmaking potential. When in Baltimore, she abandons her more liberal hat for a more conservative *sheitel*. This is especially important to her when she visits her children's schools. She explains, "I do have a *sheitel*, but I have to say that's mostly for the benefit of my children. Like if we go to Baltimore, a wedding, or some social function where I'll be around my children's friends and their families, I'll wear a *sheitel* so that I fit in better." Although she does not directly acknowledge this, as a convert, she likely also feels a certain amount of pressure to prove her *Yiddishkeit*. Hair covering is the easiest way to publicly demonstrate her level of observance.

For Vicki, her initial choice to cover her hair was also linked to her children. She explains, "My daughter had gone to Israel, and she wasn't having a very good year. So, I decided to take [hair covering] on as a *mitzvah*. I figured it would be kind of for good luck." After time, Vicki saw other benefits for her children extended from her choice to cover her hair. She is the only one of the six women who sent her children to the local public school system. They were often the only Jewish students in their grade and were certainly the only Orthodox Jews in their school. They were unable to draw on any social network established in Baltimore to find *shidduchim*. Therefore, it became even more important to Vicki that she demonstrate her family's collective level of observance through her hair covering. In a way, her actions helped to compensate for the fact that her children had not gone through the Orthodox Jewish day school system.

Haddasah's children had all completed their education before she relocated to Lancaster. Still, in her children's matchmaking processes, her hair covering played a crucial role; it retained the social ties to the Belz Hasidim for her family. She expressed a strong desire for her children to marry other Hasidic Jews and believes that her personal level of observance helped encourage this endogamy. In the case of her youngest son, who was having difficulty finding a match, Haddasah prayed while lighting Sabbath candles saying, "I don't know if this is important to you or not, but if something comes up for [my son], I will cover my *sheitel* on *Shabbos* and cover my head at night." She considered briefly rescinding this offer to God, wondering if it was really necessary to cover her hair at night. Encouraged by her son and husband, who told her "You made a promise to HaShem! Now you know! No promises to God!" Haddasah realized the power that her promise of hair covering had exerted over her family.

For the most part, the women interviewed were self-reflective about their hair covering choices. There are, however, several factors that appear to exist outside of their own awareness: a motivation to set themselves apart and identify with other observant women due to the tensions of living in a small community, a desire to have a feminized Jewish ritual, and the effect of living in a small community on their personal selection of hair coverings.

Although none of the women directly addressed the idea that hair covering served as a way of distinguishing a woman from the rest of local Orthodoxy, it appears to serve such a function. If these women lived in larger homogenous communities, the concerns that they expressed regarding perception of their observance would likely decrease. Instead, they find themselves constantly negotiating the stresses of living in an undefined community. The importance of this lack of definition is paramount. Unlike other communities—for example Williamsburg and Monsey, New York, or even Baltimore, Maryland—that imply a certain level of observance, one's *Yiddishkeit*, as a member of the Lancaster Orthodox community, could fall anywhere along the observance spectrum. With so many rituals observed privately, hair covering is the only public way that the women of Degel Israel can distinguish themselves from other less observant local Jews. It also marks them as among the more religiously observant Orthodox Jews within Degel Israel's membership.

The women's choice to cover their hair creates a cultural link between the Lancaster women and other Orthodox women. Much like Haddasah uses her hair to represent her Belz identity, the other women also use hair covering as a means of identifying with Orthodoxy at large. It functions as a demonstration of who they would be if they were not so isolated. Unlike their children, who have almost all moved away from Lancaster to settle in areas with higher Orthodox populations, the covered women of Degel Israel forge a lonely road of observance. With no general cohesion in terms of hair covering, they use their choices to represent the groups that they would associate with if their geographic situation were altered.

This self-identification process is intrinsically linked to their understanding of Jewish law. Although women in larger communities base much of their decision making process on group cohesion and social pressures, the women at Degel Israel are, in essence, left to their own devices. Although Chaya's choice as Rebbetzin could serve to role-model covering techniques, none of the women covers using her methods. Haddasah's choices are likely influenced by Belzer rabbinic decisions, but there has been no local rabbinic guidance officially provided at Degel Israel. Those who are newly observant use hair covering to signal feminized observance. As their worldview evolved, so did their external appearance. All highly educated, these women have elected, in their search for spiritual truth, to take on an external manifestation of their internal transformation. In a context that did not necessitate such a decision, social pressure cannot be blamed for their choice to cover. Rather, through their own careful consideration and evaluation of Jewish law and practice, they have made the decision to cover their hair. These women have used hair covering as an expression of feminized ritual, serving to reaffirm separate gender roles, at the same time as offering a uniquely feminine expression of spirituality.

For those women raised within Orthodoxy, hair covering represents a continued personal relationship to ritual. Although hair covering is not commonly accepted as a form of Jewish ritual observance, its practice has become more than just religious costuming. Through their daily choice to uphold and maintain the practice, these women have sacralized the act. Much in the same way that their husbands ritually lay *tefillin* (leather cases enclosing scripture written on parchment that are bound to the forehead and left arm), covering their hair is a spiritual act that embodies their continuous and daily choice of observance. Hair covering is one of the methods that they use to empower themselves within their family and community. As they seek to live out their religious commitments, covering their hair embodies their lifestyle choices. This is particularly important in Degel Israel's context, as they struggle to negotiate traditionalism in a more liberal context. Their choice to adhere to the standards established by the Orthodox communities in which they were raised rather than assimilate into the noncovering norm of Lancaster demonstrates a conscious valuing of this ritualized behavior.

When the synagogue fails to create the community that the women aspire to, they take matters into their own hands. Forced to always host social meals if they wish to eat at them (not all families at Degel Israel adhere to the same levels of kosher cooking) and working to create the type of community in which they wish their children to develop, these women are bulwarks against Orthodox assimilation. They consciously think about and engage in Jewish ritual on a daily basis. In such a small community, there is always work to be done, and they often find themselves as the voice of Lancaster Orthodoxy. Indeed, it is frequently their interpretation and application of Jewish law and ritual that defines the community. In this way their identity has become linked to ritual. Even if nonobservant Jews and secular neighbors do not recognize it, these acts of upholding ritual serve as a constant reminder of the women's nonconformist identity as "other," forcing them to be cognizant of their boundaries within both their religious and local community.

This freedom of interpretation flourishes in a small society that struggles constantly to define itself. Female hair covering is the clearest external example of this tension. When considering this, it is helpful to turn to Barbara Goldman Carrell's analysis of female head coverings presented in her article, "Hasidic Women's Head Coverings."[29] Although her investigation centers on Hasidic women, the hierarchy of hair covering that she creates seems applicable to the women of Degel Israel. Ranging from women who cover their hair with only *tichels* to women who exclusively wear human hair *sheitels*, Carrell argues that hair covering practices are concrete expressions of religious piety. In her hierarchy, the more obvious a woman's head covering (for example, a *tichel*) the more religiously observant she is. Carrell asserts that only more liberal Hasidic women cover with the less obtrusive human hair wigs. She explains, ". . . the different and ranked modes of Hasidic women's head coverings express, assert, or defend a woman's social position or level of cultural competence."[30] For Carrell, head coverings are an essential part of religious costuming and clearly represent group adherence.

The women in Carrell's study are significantly influenced by the Hasidic court with which they identify. In other words, there is relatively little autonomy involved when choosing how one covers her hair. This is, however, not the case at Degel Israel. With no standard community norm, the women are free to choose their own hair covering methods. The curious phenomenon is, despite a comparatively liberal Orthodox environment with relatively limited social control, these women have elected, for the most part, to forgo *sheitels* in favor of much more conservative *tichels*. Why would women like Kathy and Debbie, who have prominent positions in the secular community, opt not to wear a more natural looking *sheitel*? Fourth, why do the other women wear more conservative head coverings than their situation necessitates?

The answer to these questions is embedded in both the lack of community definition and the women's own perception of self. Interestingly, it is only Chaya that frequently dons a *sheitel*. This likely stems from two reasons: she was raised in an Orthodox community where wigs were the norm and, as the Rebbetzin, her level of observance is not open to the same speculation as the others. Still, she feels it important to wear more obvious head coverings when at synagogue events, suggesting that she understands the importance of her role as the female figurehead of the community.

Haddasah expresses a desire to wear an even more conservative covering than she currently does. Her daughters and daughters-in-law, however, all wear *sheitels*, despite identifying with the same Hasidic court. Her desire to wear a *shpitzel* (web-net covering often with a braid of hair across the front) may stem from a need to distinguish herself as different from the *tichel*-wearing women at Degel Israel. She describes her desire to look like other more conservative Hasidic women as follows: "With the very *Hasidische* women, I like the look. It's a very spiritual look. Now, it may not always be true, but when you look at them, you say to yourself, "Wow, she's really got it all together." Maybe you would be wrong, but a lot of women who cover that way are very very very very *tzniusdik* (modest). I admire that. I can't help it. It communicates who you are, where you are." As one of only two Hasidic women at the synagogue,[31] Haddasah's identification with the community is secondary to her affiliation with the Belz Hasidim. Were she to live in a Hasidic area, this detachment would not be necessary, as she would not have to negotiate a dual identity. By wearing the most conservative hair covering of all Lancaster Orthodox women, she publicly marks herself as the most religiously observant. In essence, her hair covering establishes a boundary between Haddasah and the rest of the Degel Israel women.

Kathy's choice to wear hats is an individual compromise. One might expect a woman with such a highly public and high powered job to opt for a *sheitel*. This would enable her to avoid questions and, if it were a high-end wig, it would most likely go completely undetected to most colleagues. Hats, on the other hand, are a more prominent reminder of difference. General American fashion is no longer a hat culture, inviting others to wonder why Kathy always wears one. Hats are, however, significantly less obtrusive than *tichels*, allowing Kathy to fully integrate hats into her professional wardrobe. They serve as a way to maintain a secular professional appearance, while still allowing for a public maker of religiosity. Unlike *tichels*, which would undercut Kathy's authority through the potential false interpretation of indicating female submission, her hats empower her to bring her private *Yiddishkeit* with her to work each day.

Debbie prefers to cover with a *tichel*; she never wears a *sheitel*, pointing out that, "It's hypocritical! Why would I cover my hair with hair that is probably more attractive than my real hair?" For her, "*Tichels* are a statement!" They represent her unapologetic commitment to living an observant lifestyle and, lest head scarves be criticized as old fashioned, Debbie proves that they can be very fashion forward. Unlike the other women who favor pre-tied *tichels*, Debbie ties her own and accessorizes them with headbands and accent scarves. She quips, "Hair covering doesn't have to be frumpy— we can still look good, just without showing our hair, you know?" She goes on to explain that by covering her hair, she is "saying to the world, 'Yes, I am an observant Jew. I'm proud of it. I don't really care what you think. Here it is!'"

Vicki and Naomi's choices appear to be equally as individualized. For Naomi, the ease of a *tichel* and its low cost is appealing. Vicki finds it unsettling to see herself not looking natural and struggles, like several of the other women, with the idea of human hair wigs may be immodest. She recounts, "The first time I wore my *sheitel* was to my daughter's wedding, and no one recognized me!" After some difficulty with obtaining a driver's license photo with a hat on, she returned wearing a *sheitel* but laments, "When I go to the grocery store or whatever, I've got this photo ID with a *sheitel*, and if my hair is sticking out or something from my hat, it's a totally different color!"

For all of the women, their hair covering choices serve to differentiate them from other women at Degel Israel. Although their hair covering patterns do not fit into Carrell's hierarchy, they have established their own based on both actual and perceived levels of observance. By wearing a prominent head covering, they differentiate and distance themselves from the less observant Lancaster Orthodoxy, as well as their secular neighbors. Chaya describes this variation eloquently, saying, "That's the beauty of *Yiddishkeit*—that we're not all one mold. Within the framework of *halakha* (Jewish law), you find where you are most comfortable. And the bottom line is that we can't judge each other. You know, that's the bottom line."

HAIR AND THE CREATION OF BOUNDARIES

It would be difficult to find an Orthodox community more diverse and yet so cohesive. Recognizing that they must embrace their lack of uniformity in order to create the social support they desire, the members of Degel Israel broach ritual creatively, allowing for a range of Orthodoxy to worship together. That said, there are external reminders of the divisions.

Like many other small synagogues, it is a daily struggle for Degel Israel to survive. Its particular location and the geographic dispersion of its members make it all the more difficult. Its members grapple constantly with the difficulty of coexisting with their Christian neighbors. Likewise, they are in a constant state of negotiation within Orthodoxy to ensure that all of their voices are heard. Although their lack of community definition causes some strain, it should not be misconstrued as an indication of apathy. On the contrary, to be a participating member of Degel Israel requires constant active engagement with one another.

Living in a cultural diaspora, one of the ways that some of the women at Degel Israel negotiate their distance from other Orthodoxy is through their head covering choices. Especially for women like Haddasah and Vicki, who no longer attend services or events at the synagogue, their sense of isolation is great. Although they have been able to create some social support online, for the most part, they travel whenever possible to be with other similarly minded Jews. The women are more or less fully integrated into the general Lancaster community, forcing them to build their social networks mainly of non-Jews. Their hair coverings serve as a way to distinguish themselves from the other women with which they work and socialize. Likewise, these same choices clearly represent the observance divisions within the synagogue.

Whether a conscious or subconscious decision, the covering women of Degel Israel do not take their hair choices lightly. It is not something that was forced on them, nor do they consider it patriarchal or oppressive.[32] For them, it is a crucial part of their self-identity and an embodiment of their spirituality. As Haddasah explains, "I find [hair covering] liberating! Going out with a covering on, except with a *sheitel* of course, does tell people, "This is what I am!" And I, yes, I like that." Their daughters, for the most part, seem to be following their mothers' lead and are covering after marriage, albeit almost exclusively with *sheitels*. With their children having largely relocated to areas with larger Orthodox populations, Degel Israel continues to actively seek new transplants to the area. Although this suggests that hair covering will continue among synagogue members, unless the community attracts a more homogenous group of new residents, the variety of hair covering techniques will persist.

This variety serves as an effective coping mechanism. It allows the women to wear three figurative hats: wherein they identify as members of their local secular community, Degel Israel, and their own strain of Orthodoxy. Their hair covering choices construct the necessary boundaries and distinctions between the women and those around them in order to enable them to create definition in a religious community that is largely undefined. Their road is sometimes lonely, and the women often feel isolated, but their adherence to hair covering demonstrates their clear attitude of antiassimilation. Indeed, it is through their intense commitment to religious ritual and observance that Lancaster Orthodoxy continues to thrive.

NOTES

1. Victoria Sherrow, *Encyclopedia of Hair: A Cultural History* (Westport, CT: Greenwood, 2006), 397; see Julia Asher-Greve, *Frauen in Altsumerischer Zeit* (Berlin, Germany: Undena, 1985); see Karen Rhea Nemet-Nejat, *Daily Life in Ancient Mesopotamia* (New York: Baker, 2001).

2. Sherrow, *Encyclopedia of Hair*, 398; Alexandra Croom, *Roman Clothing and Fashion* (New York: Amberly, 2010).

3. Sherrow, *Encyclopedia of Hair*, 398–99.

4. Sherrow, *Encyclopedia of Hair*, 399, 402.

5. Sherrow, *Encyclopedia of Hair*, 402.

6. Sherrow, *Encyclopedia of Hair*, 404.

7. Sherrow, *Encyclopedia of Hair*, 404–405.

8. Sherrow, *Encyclopedia of Hair*, 405.

9. Althea Prince, *The Politics of Black Women's Hair* (New York, Idiomatic, 2010), 57.

10. Ayana Byrd, *Hair Story: Untangling the Roots of Black Hair in America* (New York: St. Martin's Press, 2002), 44.

11. Byrd, *Hair Story*, 45.

12. See Grant McCracken, *Big Hair: A Journey into the Transformation of Self* (Woodstock, NY: Overlook Press, 1995).

13. Alfred Rubins, *A History of Jewish Costumes* (New York: Crown, 1973) 8–11.

14. Leila Leah Bronner, "From Veil to Wig: Jewish Women's Hair Covering," in *Judaism: A Quarterly Journal of Jewish Life and Thought* (Fall 1993, 465–77), 477; see also *Sefer Dat Yehudit K'hilkhata* (Jerusalem, The Committee for the Preservation of Modesty, 1973), 54.

15. See Isserles' notes to Shulhan Arukh, Orah Hayim 75:2.

16. Diane Simon *Hair: Public, Political, Extremely Personal* (New York: St. Martin's Press, 2001), 159.

17. Bronner, "From Veil to Wig," 472.

18. Chaya recalls that the only time she has intentionally left her hair uncovered was during childbirth. She had difficulty keeping a covering on during the end phase of labor and went without it. However, immediately after her children were born, she recovered her hair. Haddasah began covering her hair at night during the matchmaking process for her one son. As she

prayed for a match to be made, she offered to cover her hair even while sleeping if a good match could be found.

19. Haddasah is the only woman in this study who references regularly interacting with other Orthodox women online. The Orthodox community, at large, has been profoundly impacted by the advent of the internet and social media. There are countless blogs and websites dedicated to the art of creating beautiful Jewish hair coverings. However, the women in this study did not regularly engage with these websites. Most do not use Facebook; several do not regularly use email. Their disengagement with Orthodox online discussion forums and blogs stems from their overall decreased internet fluency.

20. Renee Kaufman, *Rachel's Daughters: Newly Orthodox Jewish Women* (New Brunswick, NJ: Rutgers University Press, 1991).

21. Association of Religion Data Archives, "Lancaster County, Pennsylvania," 2010a, http://www.thearda.com/mapsReports/reports/counties/42071_2000.asp (accessed December 28, 2010).

22. Azriela Jaffe, *What Do You Mean, You Can't Eat in My Home?: A Guide to How Newly Observant Jews and Their Less Observant Relatives Can Still Get Along* (New York: Schocken, 2005).

23. According to several of the women, Jaffe has now decided to cover her hair. One can only wonder if this is partly due to social pressure in her new community.

24. Naomi's recommitment to Judaism occurred in conjunction with moving to a different part of Baltimore and transferring synagogues.

25. Indeed, not all women who self-identify as Orthodox consider hair covering to be part of their religious identification. Although hair covering is increasing within Orthodoxy, as is exhibited at Degel Israel, not all Orthodox women uphold the practice. This is part of the reason that the women in this study feel strongly about identifying themselves as not only Orthodox but also observant.

26. Interestingly, the women separated hair covering from modesty. Although *tznius* came up in all of our interviews, the women separated modesty in clothing from their hair covering choices. Yet, despite this separation, hair covering was still interrelated with modesty, particularly when it came to which type of head covering to select.

27. Even the smallest of tasks are more difficult in such a small community. With no local kosher restaurants, if the women want to eat out, they must either eat in the kosher section of Franklin and Marshall College's cafeteria or, during the summer months, eat imbiss style food at the kosher food stand at Dutch Wonderland. Likewise, the bulk of their grocery shopping is also done in Baltimore.

28. Samuel Heilman, *Defenders of the Faith: Inside Ultra-Orthodox Jewry* (Berkley: University of California Press, 1999), 49; see Heilman 1999, 47–69.

29. Barbara Goldman Carrell, "Hasidic Women's Head Coverings" in *Religion, Dress, and the Body*, ed. Linda B. Arthur (Oxford, UK: Oxford University Press, 1999), 163–80.

30. Carrell, "Hasidic Women's Head Coverings," 174.

31. The other, a member of Chabad Lubavitch, did not respond to inquiries. When seen socially, as well as within the synagogue, she has always been observed to wear a sheitel.

32. It is true that traditional Jewish ritual is inherently male. Traditional behavior rests largely upon the assumption of gendered difference. Jewish feminists have worked to create parallel or equal rites of passage for males and females—including bris/bris bat, bar/bat mitzvah, Pidyon ha-ben/bat. However, in the case of gendered dress, how can Jewish feminists grapple with a practice that affirms gendered difference? Rather than focusing on the patriarchy out of which it grew, the real question becomes, what does it mean to traditional women today? Many Orthodox women describe modest dress as empowering. They feel that it desexualizes them, forcing society to relate to them as thoughtful individuals rather than sex objects (see Kaufman, *Rachel's Daughters*; Lynn Davidman, *Tradition in a Rootless World: Women Turn to Orthodox Judaism* (Berkley: University of California Press, 1993). The desire to be treated as a mind rather than a gendered body sounds profoundly feminist, although their traditional approach may not cleanly fit into the feminist paradigm. In this light, tradition no longer implies maleness. Rather, Orthodox women have co-opted tradition to empower themselves.

Chapter Five

Letting Their Hair Down

Orthodox Women at Degel Israel Synagogue Who Choose
Not to Cover Their Hair

My height is often one of the first things that people notice about me. As a six foot tall woman, I'm easy to spot in a crowd, have difficulty finding pants with long enough inseams, and have developed superior *sheitel* spotting abilities. From my vantage point I am able to discreetly glance down at the top of most women's heads. A good *sheitel* is difficult to detect; frequently it is only the part of the hair that deceives its wearer. When I first began attending Degel Israel Synagogue, I was not brazen enough to ask women if they were wearing *sheitels*. Usually, I could tell; although one woman did manage to slip beneath my *sheitel* radar. Having sorted the women quickly into two categories—those who cover their hair and those who do not—I was ready to proceed with my interviews. What happened next, however, surprised me.

It was the Orthodox women who chose not to cover their hair daily that complicated my research questions. I had anticipated a more cut and dry delineation between those who cover their hair and those who do not. What I discovered was that a middle group existed. It would be going too far to say that they covered part-time, just as it would be unfair to say that they never covered. These women existed in a gray area between covering and non-covering. In this chapter I will discuss both the women who choose to never cover their hair, as well as those who exist in this liminal gray area and cover their hair in certain situations, demonstrating how they use their hair to express their allegiance to the community and to the ritualized tradition of hair covering. Included in this analysis is the consideration of why women who have abandoned other acts of observant Judaism continue to engage with hair covering.

HOW IS COMMUNITY MAINTAINED? TESTING THE CONCEPT OF ADAPTED ACCULTURATION AT DEGEL ISRAEL

This chapter begins by offering an introduction to the less observant Ortho-dox members of Degel Israel Synagogue, including a discussion of adapted acculturation. Following this overview, I introduce the women interviewed to help contextualize their hair covering choices. In addition to consideration of the women's explanations of their personal motivations, this contextualized approach also considers motivations that may exist outside of their aware-ness. This serves as the basis of my analysis, which argues that these women maintain membership at Degel Israel and engage occasionally with hair cov-ering out of an interest in preserving tradition rather than a desire to adhere to strict observance. Tradition and family history function as regulators of their social behavior rather than *halakha*. Their nostalgia for past generations and for a Judaism that they view as truer and purer than Conservative or Reform practice motivates the actions described in this chapter.

As previously mentioned, the membership of Degel Israel is more diverse in terms of observance than most other Orthodox synagogues. The fact that so many levels of Orthodox observance exist within such a small congrega-tion is staggering. Yet, at the same time, such a small congregation can only continue to survive if it is open and welcoming of a variety of levels of observance. From a congregant with an Obama 2008 bumper sticker to one with a life-sized cardboard cutout of Sarah Palin, diversity expands beyond religious observance to politics, worldview, and lifestyle.

In this sense, Degel Israel is more than just a community of believers. Beyond a common basis of Judaism, the group functions more as a commu-nity of practice. As identified by Etienne Wenger, a community of practice is formed when people "engage in a process of collective learning in a shared domain."[1] Individuals may function simultaneously as participants in multi-ple communities of practice. What distinguishes them as particular members of a group is a "commitment to the domain, and therefore a shared compe-tence that distinguishes members from other people."[2] In this case, the shared domain is the synagogue, with which members elect to identify. This is, however, not enough to form community. In order to create a community, members must "interact and learn together."[3] Even without daily contact, a community can thrive based on allegiance and times of social interaction. Still, what sets a community of practice apart from a community of belief is action. A community of practice develops "a shared repertoire of resources: experiences, stories, tools, ways of addressing recurring problems—in short, a shared practice."[4] This created shared identity not only brings them togeth-er at events or activities but also forms and maintains social bonds. These bonds are crucial in the formation of community identification and serve as regulators of both community and individual behavior. As individuals increasingly identify with a particular group, their interest in shared practices or rituals increases. This intensification, in turn, increases community cohesion as well as individual attachment and identification with the group. Even when controversy arises, the negotiations that take place only heighten the sense of shared domain.

Typically religious groups are assumed to be communities of belief rather than of practice. However, Degel Israel exhibits strong traits of a community of practice. Although the central tenets of Judaism compose a shared group religious belief, the synagogue addresses shared subcultural needs which are tended to through the use of repeated rituals or customs. The needs of the congregation are not only spiritual; they are also social and function to build identity, because their Orthodox affiliation implies not only a spiritual belief but also a way of life. The congregation recognizes that it functions subculturally, and in their shared learning together, creates a community of practice that responds to the Rabbi's teaching. Indeed, the idea of learning and shared rituals functioning as personal growth is critical to understanding their importance. When viewed as an enrichment opportunity, shared practices and learning are elevated from habit and routine to a higher status of personal or spiritual development. In this light, the perceived political or lifestyle differences of Degel Israel members give way to the communal understanding of a shared domain. In this shared domain, the members of Degel Israel actively engage with their Jewishness. Although some American Jews are Jewish only in affiliation, the members of Degel Israel engage in Judaism through practice, observance, and belief. Even if community members disagree at times with what the standard of observance should be, their shared experiences help to negotiate these tensions and foster a stronger sense of domain. That is to say, if a community of practice is a group "of people who share a concern for something they do and learn to do it better as they interact regularly,"[5] the congregation is constantly learning how to better embody the characteristics of Degel Israel as they evolve and learn together to address the pressures to assimilate and forgo Orthodoxy.

Those unfamiliar with Degel Israel often question if this divide between more liberal and more conservative members is caused simply through the mixing of Modern Orthodoxy with ultraorthodoxy. This is, however, not the case. In fact, only two female congregants interviewed classify themselves as Modern Orthodox, and both women cover their hair. The majority of the female congregants, save for two Hasidic women, are not ultraorthodox. Those interviewed in chapter four tend to classify themselves as "observant." In contrast, the women in this chapter consider themselves "traditional," a distinction that is quite significant.

At present, only one book-length sociological study of Modern Orthodoxy exists, Samuel Heilman and Steven Cohen's *Cosmopolitans and Parochials: Modern Orthodox Jews in America.*[6] They consider the tensions that exist within Orthodoxy to face both outward and inward—that is to say, to exist both in and of the world. They refer to this concept as "adapted accultu-ration,"[7] an idea which they borrow from Robert Redfield's 1936 study on the process of acculturation.[8] Redfield explains that adapted acculturation is the process in which traits from both the dominant culture and subculture are melded together in order to create a cultural pattern that is a "meaningful whole."[9] Adapted acculturation allows for conflicting cultural norms to co-exist—for example, the wearing of religious dress in a secular workplace. In the case of Orthodox Jews, they, as a group, defy typical assimilation pat-terns in order to function fully as an integrated cultural group that also retains separate sets of cultural identifiers.

Heilman and Cohen's study makes the typical separation between ultraor-thodox Jewry and the rest of Orthodoxy. Those who are not ultraorthodox are considered, by Heilman and Cohen, to be Modern Orthodox. Within this group, they identify three subgroups: traditional, centrist, and nominal. They find that the group they consider to be traditional is the most observant: keeping the most stringent dietary laws, upholding the strictest observance of the Sabbath, observing even more minor fasting holidays, and having the highest synagogue attendance rates. Those who are centrist are slightly less observant: exhibiting lower rates of participation in small fasting holidays and having higher levels of abandonment of kosher cookery. Those who are nominally Orthodox are the least observant of Orthodoxy: with the lowest level of synagogue attendance and participating in more traditional ritual behavior.[10]

The importance of Heilman and Cohen's work is that it recognizes the variety within Orthodoxy, especially that there is not a strict binary separat-ing ultraorthodox and Modern Orthodox practice. However, they admit that their findings should not be used to generalize the experiences of Orthodoxy, noting that they operated from a relatively small sample to obtain their data.[11] Their results reflect what the norm is typically for most of Modern Orthodoxy, but there are marked deviations from the norm, particularly in small nonurban synagogues like Degel Israel.

Clearly a hierarchical system of observance is also in place at Degel Israel. It is difficult, however, to apply Heilman and Cohen's classification system to the congregation. The three groups that they identify—traditional, centrist, and nominal—are classified by levels of observance. In their quanti-tative study, they were able to generate statistically how closely Jewish law was followed or how strictly ritual was interpreted for various individuals. What their analysis fails to consider is the personal motivation for Orthodox affiliation and observance, something which is admittedly difficult to calcu-late.

The difficulty in applying Heilman and Cohen's classifications to Degel Israel hinges on the definition of traditionalism. For them, the more traditional an Orthodox Jew, the more observant she is. They identify traditionalists as those who are "dealing with those observances most American Jews find 'hard,'"[12] including fasting on minor holidays, keeping strictly kosher, and dedicating themselves to ritual practices. Although they did not include questions about dress on their survey, Heilman and Cohen assume that such strict observance extends to wearing the most conservative dress.[13]

After reviewing their assessment, I fully support the diversity according to observance that their classification system identifies. However, I struggle with their appropriation of the word "traditional" to equal "observant." If their system were classified on observance rather than traditionalism, it might better serve Degel Israel and other Orthodox synagogues.

The difficulty with Heilman and Cohen's hierarchy is the implication of observance as being traditional, which implies that those Orthodox Jews who are labeled "nominal" are the least interested in tradition. They consider the nominally Orthodox to be "substantially less observant than the traditionalists" and "less ritually active than the centrists."[14] They are less likely to appear outwardly Jewish through the wearing of *kippot* or *tzitzit*, observe fasting days, keep strictly kosher, and uphold other ritual observances like the *mikveh*. Furthermore, they also have the lowest attendance rate among Orthodoxy at synagogue services and are the most likely to embrace a more relaxed approach to Sabbath law. Heilman and Cohen, *Cosmopolitans and Parochials*, 64–66.[15] What makes them Orthodox is affiliation: they consider themselves more Orthodox than most other American Jews, but Heilman and Cohen consider them "Orthodox in name but not as clearly so in other respects."[16] In this hierarchy, the more observant a Jew is, the more committed she is to Orthodoxy—an equation with which I find fault. Although observance certainly demonstrates a high level of religious commitment, it does not account for spirituality or belief. This exclusion marginalizes the experiences of less observant Orthodoxy, who are, especially in small communities, a critical part of Jewish life.

Those Jews who would be considered "nominally Orthodox" at Degel Israel are those who are actually the most concerned with upholding tradition, especially in terms of creating a shared sense of cultural continuity. Unlike nominal congregants in Heilman and Cohen's study, the less observant (in terms of *kashrut*, Sabbath restrictions, the celebration of minor fasting days, and traditional dress) at Degel Israel boast high attendance rates at Sabbath services. They are among the most active in the Orthodox and local nonorthodox social community. As will be demonstrated through the interviews of the women at Degel Israel who do not engage in full time hair covering practices, their more liberal stance towards ritual and religion is filtered through their appreciation for tradition. They would balk at being called nominally Orthodox and are more likely to consider themselves traditionally Jewish rather than observant.

The tension here is between what is required by *halakha* and tradition. Some traditional behavior has been codified into Jewish law, but as can be seen throughout rabbinic commentary, Jewish law has always undergone constant reinterpretation and clarification. If typical Orthodox observance is understood to be focused on the actual laws, the understanding of traditional Judaism allows for the adaptation of Jewish practice to localities and times. Much as the *Shulchan Arukh* argues against customs replacing textual *halakha*, observant Orthodoxy focuses on the letter of the law. Traditionalists, on the other hand, are more concerned with the spirit of the law and feel freer to reinterpret it based on preference or family tradition.

For the purposes of this chapter, tradition is understood to be those expressions which are passed between generations, including but certainly not limited to beliefs, customs, rituals, and behaviors or externalizations of customs, beliefs, and rituals. Therefore, those who are most traditional are those who are most interested in preserving, disseminating, and upholding tradition. This varies from Heilman and Cohen's definition of traditionalism, which is linked to observance, or the actual enactment of traditional beliefs. That is to say, in my understanding of traditionalism is the inclusion and allowance for an appreciation for tradition that does not necessarily imply an active engagement of observance. My utilization of the word traditional, much like Heilman and Cohen's use, does not imply political views or a resistance to change. I use it to express an interest in upholding and maintaining cultural and religious continuity

SURVEYING HAIR COVERING PRACTICES

Five women are profiled in this study of women at Degel Israel Synagogue who do not engage in full time hair covering practices: Bobbie, Nancy, Rosemary, Sofia, and Susan. In addition to these women, there are at least two other women who cover their hair at temple services but not outside of the synagogue. One woman does not cover her hair, and one woman wears a wig to cover her thinning hair rather than for religious reasons. These women have not been interviewed, either because of scheduling or health reasons. Their behavior and ways in which they have described themselves to me in private conversations indicates that their motivations and beliefs are quite similar to the women profiled in this chapter.

I interviewed the five women profiled in this chapter between March and April, 2011. The women were asked a set list of thirty questions in order to establish a basis for comparison, but they were also encouraged to share personal anecdotes and opinions. Interviews generally lasted about an hour and a half, with the longest running into its third hour. Four women chose to meet in their homes, while one elected to meet in Degel Israel's library.

The women range in age from 47 to 83. All have been married, although two are widowed and one divorced. They each have between one and four children. None of their mothers covered hair consistently, and only one of their daughters covers her hair daily. All of the women are high school graduates. All of the women have attended college. Sofia holds a graduate degree, and Rosemary is in the end stages of completing a graduate degree. Susan currently is a homemaker. The other women were all employed outside of the home until retirement, and several continue to work part time or are pursuing further education. Their professions include optometry, education, nursing, informational technology, landscaping, retail, and social work.

The women's response upon being asked to classify themselves in terms of religious affiliation shows their self-perception and emic categorization regarding the importance of tradition to their Orthodox identity. One might expect that they would all, at minimum, label themselves as "Orthodox," given their affiliation with Degel Israel. Even if they were not to prefer the more specific labels of "observant" or "Torah-observant" as some of their hair covering sisters might, it would seem safe to assume that they would label themselves "Orthodox." Rather, by in large, these women struggled with how to term themselves. After careful reflection, they generally settled on the term "traditional" rather than "Orthodox."

This struggle to self-identify is significant because of its implication for what it means to be Orthodox. If these women do not self-identify as Orthodox but hold membership at an Orthodox synagogue, what does it indicate about how they understand themselves? This can be best addressed through a consideration of Erving Goffman's concept of "identity kits."[17] He argues that an individual's identity kit is critical in the presentation of self—both in terms of how the viewer and the individual react to the presentation.[18] Whether it is a tattoo or dress, body language, clothing, and hair create and maintain an image that conveys how the individual wishes to be perceived.[19]

In terms of the women at Degel Israel, hair covering and clothing function as part of their identity kit both within the synagogue and in the larger local community. The women in chapter four convey observance by consistently covering their hair more so than other presentations of self. The women in this chapter, however, have a mixed application of their identity kit. They encode their bodies and hair with different meanings based on the context. Similarly, the way that they refer to this identity varies based on context. When conversing with a non-Jew or more liberal Jew, they label themselves more readily as Orthodox, so as to convey a particular level of belief. Yet, in Orthodox circles, they struggle with terminology. Although they present an external Orthodox portrayal of identity, they are more comfortable with the phrase "traditional" to indicate their self-perception of belief and observance. They utilize their identity kit in its truest form: a supply of variables for the presentation or externalization of the perceived internal self. In doing so, they

create a middle ground of observance in which they function as totally assimilated in their daily lives and unassimilated in their religious lives.

The women share several similarities. With the exception of Susan, all of
the women are over 70 years of age. A significant difference between these
women and their general age cohort in the population is that they have had
significantly more formal education. Indeed, when looking at US Census
statistics for women over the age of 65 in Lancaster County, Pennsylvania,
only 69.7 percent have completed high school and 13.9 percent have completed a bachelor's degree or higher. Susan, who is 47 years old, falls into a
different age bracket on the Census, but still only 21.7 percent of the local
female population in her age group has completed post-high school education.[20] When looking specifically at educational levels of American Jews, 26
percent of Jews between 65–74 and 28 percent of those over 75 have completed a college degree, while 22 percent of those 65–74 and 13 percent of
those over 75 have completed a graduate degree.[21] This statistic does not
include a gendered breakdown of the percentages, but one can only assume
that Jewish men significantly outnumber their female counterparts genera-
tionally. Suffice to say that it is impressive that the women profiled in this
chapter possess such high levels of education.

In terms of religious engagement, with the exception of Susan, the wom-
en regularly attend synagogue for Saturday Sabbath services. Susan, however, is very active with the religious school programming that meets several
times during the week. Although Orthodoxy represents about 10 percent of
the total American Jewish population,[22] only about 7 percent of those over
the age of 70 identify themselves as Orthodox.[23] What is especially significant, however, is that 15 percent of American Jews over 75 and 19 percent of
those between 65 and 74 hold memberships at an Orthodox synagogue. Although about 10 percent of the Jewish population between 18 and 64 identifies as Orthodox, 24 percent hold Orthodox synagogue membership.[24] This
suggests that the struggle to self-identify as Orthodox within an Orthodox
synagogue is not unique to Degel Israel. Unlike other denominational affiliations, for example Reform Jews with which 31 percent of the 75+ population
self-identifies and where they hold 33 percent of membership,[25] Orthodox
Jews, particularly older adults, struggle to negotiate self-identification with
denominational membership.

In comparison with American Orthodoxy, the women are fairly typical in
only certain areas. 98 percent of American Orthodox Jews have inmarried,
including 100 percent of those marriages before 1970.[26] All of the women in
this chapter, save for Susan, endogamously married before 1970. Susan, who
married in 1998, is married to a non-Jew. Only 3 percent of American Orthodoxy who married during this time period married non-Jews.[27]

All of the women interviewed in this chapter will drive on the Sabbath
and are willing to do tasks that would typically be considered "work" during

Sabbath hours. Likewise, the women attend almost every Saturday morning Sabbath service. Among American Orthodoxy, only 66 percent attend religious services more than once a month.[28] Among older American Jews, synagogue attendance is significantly lower. Only 21 percent of Jews over 75 and 18 percent of Jews between 64 and 75 attend synagogue services more than once per month.[29] These percentages do not consider gender, but traditionally more Orthodox men are in attendance at Sabbath services than women, thus making it particularly paradoxical that these women boast such a high temple attendance rate.

The differences between the women stem primarily from their observance of kosher dietary laws and their views on hair covering. Eighty-four percent of American Orthodox Jews keep a kosher kitchen.[30] None of the women in this chapter keeps a fully kosher lifestyle. Only Rosemary maintains a kosher kitchen, although Nancy made a brief attempt to *kasher* her kitchen. Susan separates meat and dairy in her home but does not maintain a fully kosher kitchen. All of the women are willing to eat in restaurants and in the homes of friends.

In terms of hair covering, the women also exhibit variations in observance. Nancy only covers her hair in certain social contexts, including her son and grandson's bar mitzvahs and weddings. Susan covers her hair whenever she is in synagogue or in certain social situations like weddings or bar/bat mitzvahs. Sofia never covers her hair. Bobbie no longer covers her hair, but prior to her husband's death, she covered her hair when attending services. Rosemary fully covers her hair whenever she is attending services or learning.

HOW DOES HAIR COVERING FUNCTION AS TRADITIONAL BEHAVIOR?

Unlike the women profiled in chapter four, the women of Degel Israel who do not cover their hair on a full time basis live highly assimilated lifestyles. As I visited their homes for interviews, it was the first time that I had seen most of them out of our typical Orthodox social contexts. Although their homes were filled with Judaica, the women would, on the street at least, be indistinguishable from nonorthodox women. With the exception of Jewish jewelry, they would, in fact, be indistinguishable from non-Jews.

Not only did they look assimilated in their velour track suits and jeans, but they also lived farther away from Degel Israel. With the exception of one woman, who deliberately rents an apartment near Degel Israel so that her *shomer shabbos* son and his family can visit during the Sabbath, all of the women must drive to Degel Israel. Two of the women live in Lancaster, but the others commute between 30 and 40 minutes to worship there.

After reviewing the level of observance of the women who do not cover their hair on a daily basis at Degel Israel, two primary questions emerge: Why are these women worshipping at Degel Israel if they do not strongly identify themselves as Orthodox? How does hair covering factor into their understanding of what it means to be Orthodox or traditionally Jewish?

Before I could even ask my first question, Nancy opened our interview with, "So, before you start, I have to explain to you that I'm not really Orthodox. Well, because my background is so varied, you can't really relate me to Orthodox women. I'm at Degel because my son and his family belong to Degel." Her grandparents were Orthodox, but she was raised in a Conservative synagogue. After her family relocated when she was 13-years-old, her parents joined a Reform synagogue—the same synagogue where she would later be confirmed and married. After moving to Philadelphia, she joined a Conservative synagogue with her husband because, "that is where all of the young people were, and I wanted my children to be raised with a large Hebrew school." Finally, after careful deliberation, Nancy decides, "If I had to identify myself with a branch of Judaism, I would say Conservative."

Susan had a similar experience of sliding between the various movements of Judaism. Both of her parents were raised in Orthodox synagogues, but Susan identifies her parent's affiliation as "traditional" rather than "Orthodox." She explains, "Because I was a girl and because we lived closer to the Reform *shul*, they sent me there. They wanted me to have a Jewish education. When I became a teenager and started deciding where I wanted to go, there wasn't an Orthodox *shul* close, so I walked to the Conservative instead." When asked the branch of Judaism to which she is affiliated, she responds, "I don't identify. Even though I'm probably closer to Reform politically, I don't identify as Reform." She pauses for a moment and asks me to list a few movements within Judaism. When I reach Modern Orthodoxy, she questions what exactly Modern Orthodox means. She hesitates and responds, "Well, maybe I'm a really liberal Modern Orthodox. I mean, if I'm going to do it, I'm going to do it in the way that my family has always done it, the way I was raised. I've always leaned more towards Orthodox, but, well, you know." However, as our conversation progresses, she reconsiders her choice. She ponders, "Degel is *traditional* Orthodox. That's the kind of traditional *shul* that my grandparents grew up in and that my parents grew up in. And if I had been a boy, that's how I would have grown up. I'm comfortable here, because it feels more familiar to who I am. Degel's not the stereotype of Orthodox—they're more accepting than the rest of 'em are."

Susan's feeling of greater acceptance at Degel Israel is a generally shared sentiment. Indeed, the congregation allows for a variety of levels of observance and belief. Although Susan's choice to bat mitzvah her daughter was controversial for certain synagogue members, accommodations were made by her family, the Rabbi, and the congregation in order to create a middle ground. Rather than excluding her progressive interfaith family, Degel Israel has embraced Susan's family. They may not be stereotypically Orthodox, but their commitment to Judaism is apparent. Finally, she decides, "I think I just want to say that I'm a traditional Jew. Can we consider that a movement?"

Sofia, who still holds membership at the local Conservative synagogue, is on what she considers a spiritual path of learning more about Judaism. Part of this process for her has been worshipping at Degel Israel, where she believes the more traditional flavor is both spiritual and enriching. She anticipates transferring her membership to Degel Israel in the near future, although she plans to maintain social affiliations with the Conservative congregation through their Sisterhood. She explains, "I don't really identify with Reform at all. I don't have much Jewish education, but I just don't get Reform. To me, it just seems like the lazy man's way of being Jewish. I really think of it that way. They might as well be Protestant. But I don't think I'm Orthodox, either. I couldn't possibly be like [the Rebbetzin], with the hair covering, long skirts, and all . . . so, I guess I would be mostly Conservative, 'cause that's where I joined, and I would feel more comfortable saying that than saying that I'm Orthodox. I'm more like European Jews. They don't say they're Orthodox, but they're traditional. They just do it the right way and don't worry about labels." Indeed, only Sofia was raised outside of the United States, having fled Austria for South America at a young age, prior to her eventual relocation to the United States.

Unlike Sofia's distrust of Reform Judaism, Bobbie admits that most of her family is Reform and that she might also be Reform if it were not for her long standing affiliation with Degel Israel. She clarifies, "I would prefer, if I'm being honest, to be Reform. My daughter, she's Reform. Their kids' bar mitzvahs and everything, there is just something to be said for it. But I'm too old to change." Having been born into the congregation, her 83 year affiliation with Degel Israel is one that she is reluctant to abandon. However, when she is out of town or visiting friends and family, she seeks out a Reform synagogue at which to worship.

Only Rosemary articulated specifically that she considers herself to be Orthodox, although even she couches this statement carefully. She reports that she has "an Orthodox point of view." Later in our conversation, she rethinks this and returns to the question, explaining "I don't know if I would call myself Orthodox. Traditional, I think, is a better fit." Interestingly, only Rosemary and Sofia report having been raised as secular Jews. Rosemary specifies, "I wasn't raised in any tradition, really. My mother came from an Orthodox background, but my father was not, and it was sort of secular, I would say. In New York, it wasn't so usual to necessarily belong to a synagogue. Everyone in my [extended] family went somewhere else, but we didn't go anywhere."

Their struggle with religious self-identification begs the question of why are these women worshipping at Degel Israel if they do not strongly identify themselves as Orthodox? If they avoid using the word Orthodox to describe themselves, particularly if they consider themselves aligned with a different branch of Judaism, why attend Degel Israel or pay their membership dues? There are two other synagogues in Lancaster, Pennsylvania—a Reform and a Conservative congregation—both of which would be equidistant or even closer to the homes of these women. Likewise, nearby Harrisburg, Pennsylvania, also offers several synagogue options.

For two of the women, their choice to worship at Degel Israel is fairly self-evident. Bobbie continues to maintain membership at Degel Israel because of her longstanding family affiliation with the synagogue. Having been raised in the congregation, she feels a certain sense of belonging. Perhaps more importantly, she likely also feels a sense of legacy and responsibility. Knowing that her foremothers were instrumental in the building and development of the synagogue creates a strong sense of duty. Although she encouraged her children to seek out more liberal congregations, she is reluctant to leave Degel Israel. She explains, "I told my kids that when they got married, I said, go Reform. It's nice for the kids." Still, she feels that after an over eighty-year-long affiliation with Degel Israel, she is not ready to change. She clarifies, "You know, I was born into Degel Israel. I've always been here. I'm too old to change now."

Nancy's affiliation with Degel Israel is also not a surprise. Her son and daughter-in-law have recommitted themselves to Judaism and are now quite observant. As Nancy explained earlier, if she wishes to see them during the weekend, she needs to live within walking distance to Degel Israel and to their home, although she drives herself to both locations during the Sabbath. She admits that she feels no pressure from them to be more observant, saying, "They don't want me to be anything more than I am." However, her decision to worship at Degel Israel is clearly influenced by their religious choices.

Rosemary, Susan, and Sofia's motivation to attend services at Degel Israel is more difficult to clarify. All three women articulate that they worship at Degel Israel because of tradition. Susan believes that, "The older members of the congregation came here because, back then, you just were Jewish. It didn't matter with all of these different, you know, Reform, Conservative, Orthodox. It wasn't until much later that it mattered what kind of Jew you were. Before, you either were or you weren't. And if you were, you did it right. I like that kind of tradition." For Susan, even though she lives a highly assimilated and acculturated lifestyle, she still wants her children to experience the type of religious upbringing and worship with which she was raised. Her approach to tradition is highly nostalgic, and her primary motivation appears to be affording her children a religious experience similar to her own upbringing.

Sofia, on the other hand, does not have that same feeling of nostalgia. The worship style at Degel Israel is new to her. However, she appreciates the shift in the focus of the service towards liturgy and away from the Rabbi. One of her struggles at the local Conservative synagogue was that she did not "particularly enjoy their rabbi." Eventually she found she was avoiding services because "the Rabbi is just so egocentric." She describes this as a feeling of being lost—both spiritually and in level of interest. After studying with the Rebbetzin at Degel Israel as part of her thirst for spiritual knowledge, Sofia began attending services. She describes this saying, "I like being there [at services]. I get a certain sense of peace when I'm there. I may not know much Hebrew, but I'm learning. I know what to expect. I like the rhythm and regularity, the tradition." The way she describes her worship experience is reminiscent of a wistfulness to experience the Judaism of yesteryear. It is a Judaism that, in memory at least, is less political, more raw and pure, and, in essence, an expression of Jewishness as a way of living within a shared community.

The ritual and tradition also drew Rosemary to Degel Israel. Although she wishes that there were more social opportunities available for her, she retains her membership because, as she describes it, "I love the service. That's the reason I go. I like the ritual, the tradition. I like the things that go on in the service. I like the chanting instead of organ music. I love the Hebrew." Degel Israel also appeals to her because of the nature of the sermons. Like Sofia, Rosemary also briefly worshipped at the local Conservative synagogue. She found, however, that the sermons were "empty and lacking depth, with no real textual commentary" and that the Rabbi was "too emotional." At Degel Israel she feels like she can "experience truer religion" that is "full of tradition and history." All three women explain that the other local synagogues were too "churchy," complaining especially about the music, lack of Hebrew and liturgy, and "touchy-feely" sermons.

Clearly these women feel a strong attachment to the Judaism that they experienced in their youth. In particular, they feel strongly about the beliefs and worship styles of their parents and grandparents. If a shared appreciation for tradition serves as a unifying factor among the women of Degel Israel who do not cover their hair daily, what are their views and applications of the tradition of hair covering?

At first glance, it would seem logical that these women would completely abandon hair covering like other more traditional observances. As described in chapter four, hair covering is usually one of the last lifestyle changes that women make when becoming more observant. Why, then, do these women who have abandoned many other practices that are more commonly considered Orthodox still engage, at least partially, in hair covering? The answer seems to be twofold and overlapping: they cover their hair either as a response to social pressures to conform or out of an appreciation and respect for Orthodox tradition.

When asked if they would be willing to speak with me about hair covering, several of these women, although willing, reminded me multiple times that they would not know the "right" answers to my questions. They seemed unsure of their authority to speak about Jewish women and hair covering, because they had internalized the belief that only their more observant sisters really understood the practice. What emerged during their interviews, however, was quite different. Collectively, they were very self-reflective about their hair covering choices and were able to articulate their beliefs and decisions well. Still, they seemed largely unsure of their authority to comment on Jewish law and practice, often encouraging me to follow up with more observant congregants or the Rebbetzin for clarity. This insecurity, although completely unfounded as they always correctly articulated the very laws about which they worried, seems to be an extension of some of the tension of worshipping in such a diverse congregation. They are sensitive to the fact that, although they fully participate in synagogue life, they are still, as Heilman's hierarchy indicates, "nominally" Orthodox in comparison with other synagogue members.

Once again, this tension plays out in the form of hair covering applications. It is important to understand that none of these women reports having been directly pushed toward covering her hair. Likewise, I have never observed such actions or confrontations taking place. By and large, Degel Israel is very inclusive, at least in terms of Orthodoxy. The pressure to cover their hair is unspoken and self-perceived.

All of the women have an excellent understanding for the history and applications of hair covering, save for Sofia. During our interview, she questioned me as to why only some of the Rabbi's daughters cover their hair. She was completely unaware of the association of hair covering and marriage. She is also the only woman included in this group who has never covered her hair. This coincidence does not seem to be happenstance. Her lack of understanding of the practice presents itself in the lack of perceived social pressure to cover her hair.

For the other women, they not only more fully understand the practice, but they also perceive a certain social norm for covering their hair in particular circumstances. Although they may not feel that it is necessary to cover their hair in nonorthodox contexts, they seem acutely aware of the social norms and perceptions of hair covering. The women all report that they had an understanding for how and when to cover their hair which likely developed out of their own observation of the practices and behaviors of family and synagogue members. Although no one directly told them to cover their hair, they internalized the social norms and expectations and reacted accordingly.

Nancy, for example, covered her hair at the bar mitzvahs and weddings of her son and grandson. Although it is not surprising that she did so for her grandson, as these events took place after her son and daughter-in-law recommitted themselves to Judaism, it is notable that she covered her hair at her son's bar mitzvah. During that time her family worshipped at a Conservative synagogue. At this important life cycle event, one cannot help but wonder if Nancy's behavior is directly related to her observation of the choices made by her female family members. Her Orthodox grandmothers both donned *sheitels*. Her Conservative mother, on the other hand, always wore a hat to services. Nancy is unsure, however, if this practice was motivated by religion. She suspects it had more to do with a fashion sensibility that indicated that in order to be properly dressed, a woman wore both gloves and a hat. She shrugs, explaining, "Hats were very very very big. [My mother] had a collection of hats that was unbelievable. But she didn't just wear them to *shul*. Everyone wore hats back then."

The hat culture of which Nancy speaks is certainly true for the time period during which her mother lived. During the early twentieth century, America, along with much of the Western world, was a hat culture. Men and women were expected to wear hats when outside of the home. Hats served two purposes: in addition to sheltering the face and eyes from the sun, they evolved into status symbols that indicated socioeconomic standing and levels of perceived refinement.[31] This idea of perception is particularly important. As Fred Miller Robinson notes, because hats were significantly less expensive than other items of clothing which could convey status, they were more readily accessible to the consumer, thus more adept at "blurring and transforming . . . traditional class boundaries."[32]

Even as the wearing of hats declined, there were still certain social situations in which hats were the norm. It is not surprising that these events were highly social in nature and were ideal platforms for the display of class or refinement through hat couture. They were venues where, as Neil Steinberg quips, "Your hat is YOU."[33] In these situations, hats functioned as performative expressions of self.

This type of performance becomes blurred with religious undertones as these women describe the hat wearing patterns of their families. Much like Nancy is unsure as to whether or not her mother wore a hat to synagogue for religious reasons, Susan voices similar uncertainty. She explains, "My grandmother didn't cover her hair inside of the home, but you can't take away the fact that she was strict Orthodox. Although she always wore a hat when she went out, I don't think it was because she was Jewish. It was just a sign of the times. She grew up, you know, that's just the way you present yourself. Men always wore hats, too."

If they have an understanding that their grandmothers and mothers wore hats because of social norms and not religious obligation, why then do they cover their hair in particular social contexts? One might argue that there is a long history in both Judaism and Christianity for the socioreligious performative aspects of hats.[34] However, it is undeniable that the women of Degel Israel have an understanding of the ritualization of their hair covering practices extending beyond self-expression or performance. For them, the importance of hair covering is the ritualized tradition that it expresses.

When hair covering is viewed as both performance and ritualized behavior, it becomes clear that it functions as a "significant symbol," a phrase coined by George Herbert Mead.[35] As he explains, "the significant gesture or symbol always presupposes for its significance the social process of experience and behavior in which it arises."[36] That is to say, social interactions imbue a symbol with significance.[37] An action is given symbolic meaning through its perception and reception.[38]

The troubling aspect of hair covering as a significant symbol is in how the message of the woman is processed by the viewer. Especially in a geographical area where there are few Jewish women and even fewer that cover their hair, the meaning of hair covering is often misunderstood by the viewer. Whether it is an assumption of cancer treatment, hair loss, a fashion statement, or that the woman is a Plain Christian, the symbolic act is often falsely perceived.

Still, within the Jewish community, the choice to cover one's hair is richly symbolic. For the women who do not engage in daily hair covering, their choice to cover their hair in certain situations is all the more significant. It is a gesture to more observant synagogue members that speaks of respect. Likewise, it is an outward demonstration of an inner-commitment to tradition. This functions both to symbolically connect the wearer to Orthodoxy and to establish a figurative barrier between the wearer and less observant Jews. It shows other nonorthodox Jews that the wearer is distancing herself from the less observant and conveys her personal commitment to the legacy of Jewish tradition.

Although hair covering is considered, in its strictest sense, an extension of Jewish law, its practice has evolved into ritualized behavior. Much as Solomon Poll attributes Orthodoxy's survival to its ability to sanctify even the most secular of activities,[39] women have imbued hair covering with personal, theological, and social significance. Hair covering, when understood this way, functions dually both on the personal and social level.

Unlike the women in chapter four, who seemed relatively free from the pressures of social control, the women in this chapter sense more of an obligation to cover their hair. This distinction is critical. Those women profiled in chapter four spoke of hair covering as observance; these women view hair covering as an obligatory tradition.

This type of approach to religion is characterized in several other aspects of their religious lives. For example, although all of the women sit separated from the men by the *mechitza* during services, the women who engage in full time hair covering sit on the sides of the synagogue. The *mechitza* on the sides is fuller and virtually impenetrable by the eye. Along the back wall of the *mechitza*, however, is Plexiglas. The women of this chapter all sit along the back rows of the synagogue, affording them a full view of the service. Although they are *obligated* to sit separately, they wish to participate as fully as possible in the service. The women who consistently cover their hair, however, are more interested in upholding the actual law and not the tradition and are, therefore, more concerned with the opaqueness of the *mechitza* and its functionality.

The women's response to whether or not they feel a form of social pressure to cover their hair varies. In the case of Sofia, the only woman not to cover her hair, it is clear that she feels no social pressure. However, this is likely in large part due to her lack of familiarity with Orthodoxy. Although Nancy emphasizes that her Orthodox family does not pressure her to cover her hair, she still admits that "I can't even imagine anyone sending their [sic] child to *yeshiva* without covering their [sic] hair." She felt compelled to cover her hair at important family life cycle events, which she considers to be "traditional, just what you do in certain circles."

Similarly, Susan says she feels no pressure from her family to cover her hair, but goes on to say, "I always have known how to cover. And I've always known when to cover." Like the other women, she is very aware of what type of behavior is expected at an Orthodox synagogue. She details a visit to a Reconstructionist synagogue where she was offered a prayer shawl. With eyes wide open, she recounts, "I go Orthodox! We don't do that! Oh, no no! Whew! No, I can't! We don't do that, no no no!" She goes on to say, "And women wearing *kippot*? Ridiculous. I won't even wear slacks into the *shul*. There are just certain things [you don't do], you know, out of respect."

Of the women, Bobbie seems the most critical of hair covering. Although she covered her hair at services after marriage, she points to her heart and explains, "In my opinion, it's not what's covered. It's what's in here that counts. You can be covered and not be such a good person." Likewise, she is the only woman who mentions that some women cover their hair with *kippot*, and that she considers this an acceptable hair covering.

Bobbie's mistrust of hair covering as being indicative of a good Jew is one shared by several of the women. She articulates this tension, saying, "I look at [the more observant members of the congregation] and I say, if that's religion, being so critical of other people, then I don't want to be religious. I just feel like, when you're real religious like that, some of them are not nice to people. And I don't think that's religion. You gotta treat everybody the way you want to be treated and see good in everyone." Unlike the women in chapter four, who spoke more about the hardships of living observantly in a small community, these women spoke more openly about the difficulty of living as a *Mensch*, a humane person. Nancy points to her heart and says, "My Jewishness is in here . . . I feel like I have always lived a moral life. And I think that is what Judaism is. They want you to be moral. They want you to be charitable . . . I don't feel like I have to have a kosher home [in order to be a good Jew], but that's not saying I'm right." Susan agrees, sharing, "But I was like, you want to be respected for being Jewish, you wanted to be respected for this Orthodox view point, so why can't you respect my view-point? That's my attitude. If you want respect, you need to give it to others. You may not agree with it, but you have to be open to that [sic] it's their choice. I don't think anyone is forcing anyone to be a certain way. It's a choice that they [sic] made."

Despite assuring me that they feel no external pressure to cover their hair from other synagogue members, it is clear that these women put a certain degree of pressure on themselves to conform. This self-regulatory pressure likely stems from a desire to fit in and, not surprisingly, is an extension of their emphasis on tradition.

Although they may feel no direct pressure to heighten their levels of observance, indirect pressure is still at work. They are aware that, although they may dine in the homes of other congregants, they cannot entertain them in their own homes. Likewise, they may help prepare food at the synagogue, but they cannot prepare food in their own homes to share at social events.

Similarly, after parking on the Sabbath on the back gravel lot that is beyond the actual synagogue parking lot, they stash their car keys discretely in a pocket or on a shelf in the coat room. None elects to carry a purse into the synagogue, although each would carry one elsewhere during the Sabbath. In other words, these women are aware of the social and religious norms at Degel Israel and adapt in order to comply.

The women at Degel Israel engage in hair covering much the same way. Although Sofia does not cover her hair during services and has never felt any pressure to do so, the other women have a sense of obligation to cover their hair. They feel this, at minimum, at large social events and, for several, at all times within the synagogue. This action is highly performative; it demonstrates to the viewer that the woman is a more traditional Jew who aligns herself with Orthodoxy. Moreover, it is an externalization of the wearer's desire to be considered a serious Jew. Through covering her hair, she demonstrates her commitment to upholding traditional Judaism. Not only does it help her fit in with other Orthodox women, but it reaffirms the wearer's dedication to both religious and social aspects of Jewish tradition.

Prior to our interviews, I had expected that I would hear the most conservative rhetoric from the most observant women and would hear more feminist rhetoric from the women who did not cover their hair daily. What I found, however, was the exact opposite. Those women who covered their hair full time spoke of agency, empowerment, and self. The women in this chapter, however, had a rhetoric of tradition. Even when they did not use the word, they alluded to traditional behavior and family legacy. Their interviews were peppered with stories of their parents and grandparents, especially when speaking about behaviors that were important to them or why they continued to worship at an Orthodox synagogue.

The women all worried about the future of Judaism, more so than the women in chapter four. Despite having married a non-Jew, Susan worries about her teenage daughter not meeting Jewish teens to date. She explains, "I'll support my kids no matter how they go. But I want them to have a Jewish lifestyle, like me, like my parents, my grandparents." Bobbie voices a similar desire for future generations to continue to develop the respect that was instilled in her. She worries, "Everything is so different today. You know, when I was younger, whether it was a doctor or a rabbi or a teacher, you showed respect. People aren't like that anymore. Respect is missing from the newer generations. My dad always told me, Judaism is in here [puts hand on heart]. You gotta treat everybody the way you want to be treated. He pounded that into us kids when we were little. And that's right! And nobody had a cruel word about my dad, 'cause he never, never had a mean word to say about anyone. He saw good in everyone."

The one way in which these women straddle the paradigm of feminist versus traditional rhetoric is when they speak about Jewish education. They expressed a universal sadness that they had not received greater Jewish education in their youth. They have all ensured that their daughters were given ample opportunities to learn. In fact, some of them have even bat mitzvahed their daughters. In addition, they have taken steps to further educate themselves. Only Rosemary remains in the sanctuary during the chanting of the Torah portion; not coincidentally, she is the only one with strong enough Hebrew skills to fully follow along. The rest of the women retreat to the synagogue library, where they study together with the Rebbetzin. They have taken hold of their own education and are quite progressive in their desire to expand their Jewish learning. That said, their primary concern still seems to be tradition. During their weekly study sessions, conversation is equally divided between the struggle to live as a Jew in Lancaster County and the fears that they have about the abandonment of tradition.

It would be an inaccurate generalization to assume that these women are focused on the past because of their advanced age. Surely their age does influence their mindset and beliefs, but they are, as a whole, quite progressive. Their interest in tradition is not in a stale and old world sense of traditionalism. Rather, they have a strong sense of Jewish women as responsible for the survival of future generations of Judaism. Although they may struggle with the need to live highly observant lives, they see value in the legacy of Judaism. As Bobbie clearly sums it up, "My mom and grandmother were great women—both as Jews and as people. Why wouldn't I want me and my daughter to be like them?"

KEEPING THE FLAME ALIVE

Orthodox Jews are struggling to negotiate the tensions of assimilation and acculturation. The shift or, as some would see it, schism between Modern Orthodoxy and ultraorthodoxy is becoming ever more pronounced.[40] What is particularly interesting is how this tension plays out under one shared roof at Degel Israel Synagogue. Surely these two groups would have subdivided if the geographical situation were altered; yet, in Lancaster, they are completely dependent on one another.

These women may struggle to call themselves Orthodox, especially when they perceive themselves to be considerably "less Orthodox" than more observant members of the congregation. Yet, without their dedication and, to be frank, monetary support, the synagogue would falter. They are an integral and crucial part of the community.

Their approach to Orthodoxy should not be labeled as "nominal." They are just as engaged in their Jewishness as other more observant synagogue members. They are actively involved in synagogue life, seek out countless Jewish educational opportunities, and are extremely active in local volunteer work. They speak more about their personal spirituality and strong desire to uphold tradition as opposed to the women of chapter four who speak more about observance. For much of the local community, these women are the face of what it means to be an assimilated Jew who concurrently upholds traditional beliefs.

This active engagement with tradition that functions alongside of contemporary acculturated lives is the essence of what it should mean when we speak of Modern Orthodoxy. However, the phrase is now typically used to refer to observant Jews who are not ultraorthodox. It is no wonder that these women struggle to classify themselves. Their own classification of "traditional" articulates well their approach to Judaism. It is filled with an appreciation for the past and attempting to honor the legacy of their foremothers, they face forward and fully live in the world while trying to keep the flame of tradition alive for future generations.

NOTES

1. Etienne Wenger, "Communities of Practice," 2011, http://www.ewenger.com/theory (accessed June 20, 2011); see Etienne Wenger, *Communities of Practice: Learning, Meaning, and Identity* (Cambridge, UK: Cambridge University Press, 1998); see Etienne Wenger and

Jean Lave, *Situated Learning: Legitimate Peripheral Participation* (Cambridge, UK: Cambridge University Press, 1990).

2. Wenger, "Communitites of Practice."

3. Wenger, "Communitites of Practice."

4. Wenger, "Communitites of Practice."

5. Wenger, "Communitites of Practice."

6. Samuel Heilman and Steven Cohen, *Cosmopolitans and Parochials: Modern Orthodox Jews in America* (Chicago: University of Chicago Press, 1999).

7. Heilman and Cohen, *Cosmopolitans and Parochials*, 1–18.

8. Heilman and Cohen, *Cosmopolitans and Parochials*, 1–18.

9. Heilman and Cohen, *Cosmopolitans and Parochials*, 152.

10. Heilman and Cohen, *Cosmopolitans and Parochials*, 60–61.

11. Heilman and Cohen, *Cosmopolitans and Parochials*, 33–37.

12. Heilman and Cohen, *Cosmopolitans and Parochials*, 58.

13. Heilman and Cohen, *Cosmopolitans and Parochials*, 29.

14. Heilman and Cohen, *Cosmopolitans and Parochials*, 64.

15. Heilman and Cohen, *Cosmopolitans and Parochials*, 64–66.

16. Heilman and Cohen, *Cosmopolitans and Parochials*, 66.

17. Erving Goffman, "Identity Kits," in *Dress, Adornment and the Social Orders*, ed. M. Roach and J. Eicher (New York: John Wiley and Sons), 246–47.

18. Erving Goffman, *Asylums: Essays on the Social Situation of Mental Patients and Other Inmates* (New York: Anchor, 1961), 21–22.

19. Goffman, *Asylums*, 14–21; Erving Goffman, *The Presentation of Self in Everyday Life* (New York: Anchor, 1959).

20. US Census, "Lancaster County Pennsylvania: Educational Attainment," 2011c, http://factfinder.census.gov/servlet/STTable?_bm=y&-geo_id=05000US42071&-qr_name=ACS _2009_5YR_G00_S1501&-ds_name=ACS_2009_5YR_G00_&-redoLog=false (accessed May 16, 2011).

21. Miriam Rieger, *The American Jewish Elderly* (New York: National Jewish Population Survey, 2004), 8.

22. United Jewish Communities, "National Jewish Population Survey 2000–01: Orthodox Jews: A United Jewish Communities Presentation of Findings," 2004, http://www.jewishdatabank.org?Archive?NJPS2000_Orthodox_Jews.pdf (accessed June 24, 2011), 6.

23. Rieger, *The American Jewish Elderly*, 17.

24. Rieger, *The American Jewish Elderly*, 17.

25. Rieger, *The American Jewish Elderly*, 17.

26. Jonathon Ament, *American Jewish Religious Denominations* (New York: National Jewish Populations Survey, 2005), 30.

27. Ament, *American Jewish Religious Denominations*, 30.

28. Ament, *American Jewish Religious Denominations*, 30.

29. Rieger, *The American Jewish Elderly*, 16.

30. Ament, *American Jewish Religious Denominations*, 30.

31. See Hilda Amphlett, *Hats: A History of Fashion in Headwear* (New York: Dover Publications, 2003), 156–175; Diana Crane, *Fashion and Its Social Agendas: Class, Gender, and Identity in Clothing* (Chicago: University of Chicago Press, 2000), 82–87.

32. Crane *Fashion and Its Social Agendas*, 82; see Fred Miller Robinson, *The Man in the Bowler Hat: Its History and Iconography* (Chapel Hill: University of North Carolina Press, 1993), 39–40. Robinson's treatment of hats is almost exclusively male, but his work represents an important understanding of how hats function socially.

33. Neil Steinberg, *Hatless Jack: The President, the Fedora, and the History of American Style* (New York: Plume, 2004), 131.

34. See Michael Cunningham and Craig Marberry,*Crowns: Portraits of Black Women in Church Hats* (Ann Arbor: University of Michigan Press, 2000).

35. George Herbert Mead, *Mind, Self, and Society* (Chicago: University of Chicago Press, 1934).

36. Filipe Carreira da Silva, *G. H. Mead: A Critical Introduction* (New York: Polity, 2007), 35.

37. Mead, *Mind, Self, and Society*, 46–49.

38. George Herbert Mead, *The Philosophy of the Act* (Chicago: University of Chicago Press, 1938), x–xi.

39. Solomon Poll, *The Hasidic Community of Williamsburg: A Study in the Sociology of Religion* (New York: Free Press, 1962).

40. See Samuel Heilman, *Defenders of the Faith: Inside Ultra-Orthodox Jewry* (Berkley: University of California Press, 1999).

Chapter Six

Flipping Their Wigs for Judaism

Nonorthodox Women Who Choose to
Cover Their Heads

My mother sent me an email that included the following, "Pat and I were at the deli today. The woman sitting at the table next to us had on a *yarmulke*. I should probably know the answer to this by now, but what kind of Jew was she?" My mother has humored me by listening to my frequent hair and head covering musings and has become quite adept at identifying *sheitels*, *tichels*, snoods, and hats. She was right to question why a woman would be wearing a *kippah* (Hebrew for cap, the traditionally male Jewish skullcap; also known as *yarmulke* from the Yiddish) in public. She had seen them worn during religious services, but, in a deli, it seemed strikingly out of place.

I wish that I could speak with this woman and ask her about her choice to wear a *kippah*. Indeed, her decision to cover her head, especially outside of the synagogue, is a bold choice made by very few Jewish women. Much like their male counterparts, relatively few nonorthodox Jews cover their heads outside of the synagogue. Furthermore, fewer women than men cover their heads at services. The woman covering her head in the deli defies both of these stereotypes, leading viewers—like my mother and her friend—to wonder what message she was conveying through her head covering.

It is important to understand the difference between head and hair covering. When a Jewish woman covers her hair with a hat, *sheitel*, or *tichel*, she is trying to ensure that the majority of her hair is privatized and out of view; she does so only after marriage. Head covering's purpose, on the other hand, is not to conceal all of the hair, but rather to ensure that the head is covered in some way. Although this can be done through the wearing of traditional hair coverings (*tichel*, *sheitel*, snood, or hat), it is more common to wear a *kippah*.

97

Both married and unmarried women cover their heads. If head and hair covering are understood to be distinct practices, how are they similar or different? And do the women who engage in these practices have the same motivations?

AMERICAN JEWISH HEAD COVERING PRACTICES

In this chapter I will begin by offering pertinent background information on the wearing of *kippot* and of Jewish women's appropriation of the practice. I will then introduce the women interviewed, explaining both their similarities and differences. In my analysis of their beliefs and behaviors, I argue that although there are similarities between head and hair covering, the critical differences between the two practices are the emphasis on egalitarianism and the affirmation of the religious rights of Jewish women.

Of all Jewish practices and beliefs, one of the practices that Americans seem to be most familiar with is the wearing of *kippot* (pl. from Hebrew, singular *kippah*). These head coverings are typically worn by Jewish men—either alone or under a hat—and are both a constant reminder of their religious dedication and an external announcement of their religious or cultural affiliation. *Kippot* differ from hats in several ways. Hats typically have a crown and a brim and cover most of the head. *Kippot*, on the other hand, are essentially caps. They are brimless, sit closer to the head, and do not cover the entire head. Unlike hats, which sit on the head, *kippot* conform to the head.

Much as female hair covering is not biblically mandated, male head covering is also considered *minhag* (cultural). Codified throughout the Talmud and rabbinic texts,[1] men are told to, "Cover your head in order that the fear of heaven may be upon you."[2] Although there are no artistic renderings of Jewish costuming before 1000 CE, it is widely accepted that early Jewish costuming included mandatory head covering for both men and women.[3]

Artistic depictions of Jewish men from the early twelfth century on indicate that *kippot*—or at least some form of male head covering—are consistently factored into Jewish male attire. It would not be until the late thirteenth century that the Zohar would mention that Jewish men should cover their heads during prayer. However, earlier letters and texts refer to the importance of not praying bareheaded. By 1646, the *Turei Zahav,* a commentary on the *Shulchan Arukh*, remind Jewish men that their head covering is critical, as it distinguishes them from non-Jews. Medieval Jews would largely base their head covering choices on the social norms of the lands in which they lived. Many times they were forced to wear a *Judenhut* (from German, literally a Jew-hat) to publically identify and stigmatize them as Jews when they were outside of the ghetto walls. By the end of the eighteenth century, the Vilna

Gaon (a prominent Jewish leader) ruled that men should cover their heads as a sign of respecting the Divine. He explained that if men were only required to cover their heads during prayer, by continuously covering their heads, they demonstrated an increased level of religious commitment and piety.[4]

In contemporary practice, *kippot* exhibit a strikingly similar trajectory to women's hair covering. Historically *kippot* served as an external marker of religious affiliation. After the great wave of Jewish immigration to the United States (1880–1920), Jews for the first time had the choice of whether or not they wished to affiliate with Judaism. That is to say, in the United States, they were no longer legally identified as Jewish in identity papers and passports; instead, their Judaism was a religious or cultural choice. Many men and women abandoned external markers of their Jewishness, favoring a more assimilated American fashion style. The first generation of American-born children reached adulthood during or after the interwar years. Having never experienced life in Eastern Europe, with pressure to assimilate from their parents, and their own desire to be truly Americanized, traditional clothing (*tzitzit*, caftans, *shtreimels*) and headgear (*kippot*, *tichels*, *sheitels*) were only worn by the most religiously observant.

After immigration, more pious Jews attempted to transplant their rituals and practices in their entirety. Rather than assimilating, they wished to continue to live as they did in Eastern Europe—separate and distinct. The promise of America, for these observant Jews, was the economic freedom to have earning potential while still retaining a religious lifestyle. The assimilation and secularization that they witnessed prompted Rabbi Jacob David Wilowsky to admonish American Jews in 1900 that, "It was not only home that the Jews left behind in Europe. It was their Torah, their Talmud, their *yeshivot*—in a word, their *Yiddishkeit*, their entire Jewish way of life."[5] Word spread quickly back to Eastern Europe that America provided not only economic opportunity but also significant religious danger. Those concerned with this, however, were among the minority of immigrants.

Unlike the pious Jews who were willing to take lower paying jobs in order to fully participate in the Sabbath and other Jewish holidays, most Jewish immigrants focused on economic success, for which they were willing to sacrifice Jewish observance, including religious dress. Although the majority of immigrants were interested in self-identifying as Jewish, they attempted to merge a fully assimilated American lifestyle with their religious beliefs. The difficulty, however, was twofold. First, it was extremely difficult to observe religious holidays and the Jewish Sabbath, which lasts from Friday evening through Saturday nightfall. Many Jewish men found themselves faced with both willingly and unwillingly working on Saturdays. As Jonathan Sarna aptly describes the situation: "They struggled, in short, to find some balance between their ancient faith, their economic aspirations, and their utopian ideologies—a halfway covenant between tradition and change."[6]

If they were willing to compromise on the observation of the Sabbath and of Jewish holidays, it is no surprise that Jewish spirituality, as well as the role of individual Jews in both religious obligation and religious community, significantly changed between 1920 and 1945. American Jews were not forced to legally identify themselves as Jewish, allowing their affiliation with Judaism to be both personal and voluntary. Coupled with the profound deficit of rabbis, which caused a severe lack of Jewish leadership, the increasing privatization of Judaism into the home produced a drastic schism within the Jewish community. There were Jews who went to *shul* (Yiddish for synagogue) and were largely isolated from both the American and Jewish community, and then there was the majority of American Jewry who had replaced active participation in synagogue life with American culture. By 1900, the *American Jewish Yearbook* estimates that 80 percent, or four out of five, American Jews no longer actively participated in a synagogue.[7] Sarna calculates, using 1906 Census data, that only 26 percent of American Jews could have even been seated within American synagogues; that figure translates into 364,700 seats for 1.4 million Jews. In contrast, American churches of the same time could seat about 70 percent of the American Christian population. This figure would decrease by the 1916 Census; Sarna estimates that only 12 percent of American Jews were included on synagogue membership rosters[8] meaning that possibly even fewer were attending services but retained membership through the paying of dues.

In the *shtetls* of Eastern Europe, Jews had lived as a racialized "other" to the Christian majority. Whether it was their lifestyle, religious beliefs, eating habits, or dress, they existed on the periphery of their community. Relocated to the United States, they now had the option of fully integrating into American life. One of the first ways in which they could assimilate was through clothing. Even if the language barrier kept them from interacting with their neighbors, they could, at minimum, "look American." Likewise, in pursuing their economic dream, men were quick to replace "Old World" clothing with contemporary American fashion, in order to blend in with their American work colleagues and market themselves as fully American to their neighbors.

As Jewish dress became virtually indistinguishable from American fashion, so too did Jewish headwear. In keeping with American hat culture trends, men and women appeared with their heads covered until after World War II. However, it was only the most pious of Jewish men who wore *kippot* underneath their hats. When American men began appearing in public bareheaded, so too did American Jewish men. *Kippot* were only worn daily by the most religiously observant. Other Jewish men either abandoned head covering completely or only wore *kippot* when in the synagogue. Although male head covering would experience a revival in Israel after the Yom Kippur War (1973) when wearing *kippot* became a symbol of national pride, their popularity did not transfer to the United States.

The importance of what a *kippah* communicates is often lost on those who are not familiar with the caps. There is a seemingly endless list of variations from *kippot* emblazoned with athletic team logos to traditional black velvet *kippot* or multicolored crocheted *kippot*. The *kippah*, much like Jewish women's hair covering, is both a fashion and a religious statement. *Kippot* styles vary between *Ashkenazic* (Jews with German and Eastern European roots) and *Sephardic* (Jews with Spanish and north-African roots) Jews. Not only can they mark cultural affiliation, but *kippot* are also often a political statement. As Eli and Elise Davis explain, ". . . the [male] head covering has, for many, taken on the significance of a badge . . . [men] covering their head has become significant and valuable, not because it has any inherent meaning but rather as conventional sign of belonging to a certain group of people and of commitment to a certain way of life."[9] The clearest example of this is the *kippah sruga*, a popular crocheted style. Within Israel, this style of *kippah* is strongly associated with religious Zionism. However, in the United States it is less political and usually indicates affiliation with the Reform or Conservative movements.[10] Furthermore, *kippot* can also indicate level of religious observance; for example, velvet *kippot* are typically associated with Orthodoxy, particularly if they are black.

The other thing that has historically been encoded in *kippot* is maleness. Historically head covering has been male in contrast to hair covering, which has traditionally implied femininity. American Jewish feminism took shape in the 1970s. Early issues included the exclusion of women from *minyanim* (pl. *minyan*, the quorum of ten men required for certain religious events and rituals), divorce rights, and the involvement of women in Jewish ritual.[11] Also included in this move toward religious egalitarianism, Jewish feminists broached issues surrounding the ordination of female clergy, the full participation of women in synagogue life, allowing women to read from the *bimah*, and in the role of the Jewish woman both at home and in the community.[12] Often overlooked in this struggle are the ways in which head covering factored into Jewish feminism and how women, even those who do not label themselves feminist, religiously fashion their bodies. If Jewish men cover their heads out of respect for the Divine and as a sign of their religious commitment, can (or should) Jewish women do the same?

JEWISH WOMEN WHO COVER THEIR HEADS

Six women are profiled in this study of women in Central Pennsylvania who cover their heads: Beth, Carla, Ella, Hope, Rachel, and Suzanne. In addition to these women, one additional woman, Becky, will also be referenced. Although she was not formally interviewed, her comments come from private e-mail communication in which she answered the same set of interview questions. I interviewed these women during July, 2011. They were asked a set list of thirty questions in order to establish a basis for comparison, but they were also encouraged to share personal anecdotes and opinions. Interviews generally lasted about forty minutes to one hour. Three of the women chose to meet in local eateries, two in their home synagogues, and one in her home.

It is not surprising that no women at Degel Israel cover their heads with *kippot*—the practice is decidedly unorthodox. The seven women profiled in this chapter all worship at other local synagogues in Central Pennsylvania. Four of the women self-identify as Reform; three consider themselves Conservative. Two admit that if they lived in a different locale, they might affiliate with a Reconstructionist synagogue.

The women range in age from 27 to 72. Four of the women are married; two are divorced; and one is living in a long-term committed life partnership and would marry if she legally had the right. Five of the women have children; two of the women are childless.

Like the Orthodox women interviewed, these women are also highly educated. All seven of the women have attended college, although only six completed their degrees. Two of the women have pursued additional coursework or certificate programs—including, courses through Gratz College. Likewise, Hope, Carla, Ella, and Suzanne have all completed graduate degrees. In fact, Suzanne has completed two graduate degrees, and Carla has completed a remarkable three master's degrees. The women work in a variety of jobs. All are currently employed, except for Ella who retired just days before our interview. Professionally they work as a communications analyst, an administrative assistant, a teacher, a social advocate, a cantor, a cantorial soloist,[13] and a rabbi.

All of these women cover their heads in some form. Only Carla covers her head constantly. Beth and Becky frequently cover their heads outside of the synagogue. Hope, Ella, and Suzanne all cover their heads when at synagogue, at other religious events, or in Jewish social contexts. Rachel is ambivalent about her head covering practices and does not cover her head consistently. She understands why head covering is important to some women, but is unsure if it "agrees" with her. *Kippot* "feel masculine" to her, and she desires the practice to feel "female-affirming." Because of this tension, she struggles to negotiate her desire to feel feminine with a practice she sees as steeped in masculinity. The types of *kippot* used by the women are as unique as they are. Varying from "feminized" wire crocheted *kippot* to "masculine" *kippot sruga*, the women base their head covering choices on many factors, including comfort, fashion, color, head size, and political implications.

In terms of religious observance, the women are highly engaged in Jewish life both in the synagogue and at home. All regularly attend Sabbath services. Most are involved in their synagogue's Sisterhood and participate in other local Jewish social groups, events, and educational opportunities. Only Carla lays *tefillin*, although Beth indicated she is interested in pursuing the practice. All but one of the women regularly wears a *tallis* when worshipping. Four women keep a kosher kitchen; three women do not.

One striking element that emerged during my interviews was that four of the seven women have converted to Judaism. Three of the seven women, including two who converted to Judaism, are clergy. In creating my interview pool I did not specifically seek out members of either group; therefore, it was particularly noteworthy to discover these two trends. There are relatively few women in Central Pennsylvania synagogues who cover their heads. When the women were asked how many other women at their synagogues covered their hair, they typically identified between zero and five others, often unknowingly naming other women I had interviewed.

DISTINCTIONS AND OVERLAPS BETWEEN HEAD AND HAIR COVERING

The line between head and hair covering is complicated. On the one hand, the motivations behind the two practices are fundamentally different. Yet, at the same time, their applications are sometimes indistinguishable. Even when discussed, the terms head covering and hair covering are often used interchangeably. In particular, nonorthodox Jewish women in Central Pennsylvania, including those interviewed and women with whom I am acquainted, frequently use hair covering as a synonym for head covering. This suggests a manifestation of the tension caused by living as an extreme minority. Central Pennsylvania is home to an extremely concentrated population of Anabaptist Christians including Amish, Old Order Mennonites, and conservative Brethren. These women also engage in hair covering, and it is commonplace to see women wearing white or black prayer coverings or bonnets. The Plain community and much the general population refer to these as "head coverings," regardless of size or form.[14] Local Jewish women, therefore, feel uncomfortable identifying their practices as "head covering" because of the Christian implications. Rather, by saying "hair covering," they align with their Orthodox sisters and distinguish themselves from other local Christian women who cover their hair. Despite comingling the two phrases, these women who cover their heads understand their practice to be fundamentally different than Orthodox hair covering. Because of this and to help maintain clarity, I refer to hair covering as the Orthodox practice of entirely covering the hair and consider head covering the practice of donning *kippot*.

Another point of terminology that is important to address is the use of *kippah* versus *yarmulke*. Technically the two words are interchangeable and mean the same thing. However, unlike *tallis/tallit* or *Shabbos/Shabbat*, which the women freely alternated between Yiddish and Hebrew forms, they almost never used the word *yarmulke*. This surprised me, as I expected a preference for the Yiddish form, especially given the acceptance of *yarmulke* into American vernacular. At first I considered that the women's preference for the Hebrew might stem from their lack of Yiddish fluency. Indeed, none of the women was raised or currently lives in a Yiddish speaking home. However, they showed proficient Yiddish knowledge in the other terminology they utilized, which belies this theory.

In reviewing transcripts of their interviews, I was struck by an unintentional differentiation the women made. Each time they used the word *yarmulke*, they were referring to men or to non-gendered hair coverings, for example, "The *yarmulke*s given out at a wedding." When discussing their own head coverings, they used "*kippah*"—a word that they rarely used when referring to male or non-gendered head coverings, unless making a direct comparison to their own choice. For example, "My *kippah* is smaller than the *kippot* most men wear, because my head is smaller."

The women seemed unaware of their rhetorical choice. By using the less colloquial Hebrew, they establish a gendered differentiation. In doing so, they claim the practice for themselves. As Jewish feminists work toward evolving traditional rituals and practices to be more egalitarian, this has caused not only a cultural but also a rhetorical shift. Just as bar mitzvahs are for boys, bat mitzvahs are for girls. If male babies are circumcised during a *bris*, female infants are named during *bris bat*. The first born son is redeemed during *Pidyon Ha-ben*, and the first born daughter may be redeemed either through *Pidyon Ha-bat* or a *Simchat Bat*. Therefore, it is no great surprise that this gender parallelism extends to head covering. If Jewish men wear *yarmulke*s, Jewish women wear *kippot*. The practice is equal, but the rhetorical shift indicates its break with tradition.

This same differentiation does not occur when referring to prayer shawls, which the women referred to interchangeably as *tallitot* and *tallisim*.[15] Although they are also traditional religious garb, they are not defined as "Jewish *male* prayer shawls" the same way that *yarmulke*s are typically defined as "skullcaps worn by Jewish *men*." *Tallisim* may also be traditionally worn by men, but the word itself is not embedded with masculinity the same way as yarmulke.

By using the word *kippah* to refer to their head covering, the women claim both the practice and the material object for themselves. Although they view the practice as egalitarian, their choice to cover their heads is bold and uncommon. In a religion where even many men appear bareheaded, laying claim to the practice and establishing it as a Jewish woman's right is more than a rhetorical shift. It alters the paradigm of how nonorthodox Jewish women externalize and embody their faith.

The women interviewed in this chapter are acutely aware of how their choice to cover their heads is unconventional. Likewise, they all agree that head covering is fundamentally different than hair covering. There are, however, more similarities between the two practices than the practitioners might expect. There are three primary ways in which the head and hair covering are similar: the feminist rhetoric which the women use when speaking of their choices, their active engagement in the practice, and their externalization of *Yiddishkeit*.

The practice of head covering is frequently associated with feminism. Therefore, I was surprised that of the seven women interviewed, two of the women do not consider themselves feminists, and one carefully cases her self-description, saying, "I guess, if pressed, I would say I'm a little bit feminist, but not ultrafeminist." This labeling is also not a generational difference. Indeed, it was the older women interviewed who were more likely to self-identify as feminists.[16]

Despite their mixed acceptance of the feminist label, the Orthodox women nonetheless employ feminist rhetoric to describe their decisions and practices. Hope, tucking her waist length blonde hair behind her ears, explains, "There is no mistaking my intent when you look at my *kippah*." Despite her slight stature, Carla's presence commands respect. She describes head covering as, ". . . part of my self-agency. I get to call the shots." Even Rachel, who most strongly opposed labeling herself a feminist, points out, "I don't think that any decision or choice that a woman legitimately makes for herself could be considered anti-woman. If she wants to do it, she's pro-woman. Pro-herself."

Intent. Agency. Anti-woman. Pro-woman. Choice. These same phrases are used by the Orthodox women who cover their hair. For both groups of women, their choices are intentional, carefully implemented, and part of how they conceptualize themselves as gendered religious bodies. Unlike the women at Degel Israel who do not cover their hair daily or other Jewish women who do not wear *kippot*, these women speak of their headwear in terms of conscious choices about self-identity.

This understanding of agency translates over into another similarity between the two groups of women: their active engagement in the practice. Each time a woman covers her hair or her head, she makes a choice to uphold the tradition. Beth, with short cropped hair and boxy clothing, explains, "I love [to cover my head] and the feeling that it gives me." Carla pounds her fist on the table as she emphasizes, "When I don't have my head covered, I feel naked, like I'm not wearing a bra or not wearing clothes!" The experiences of women who cover their heads or hair are remarkably similar. They recall the first time they covered; they describe the feeling of choice that they experience each time they go from bareheaded to covered; and they illustrate the methods with which they choose their coverings using strikingly similar language.

Whether it is the selection of a hat, *tichel*, *sheitel*, snood, or *kippah*, the women tend to base their headwear selection on the same three factors: style, function, and context. In terms of style, many of the women speak of matching their covering to their outfit. Much like Orthodox women speak of selecting a hat or *tichel* based on color or fashion style, women who cover their heads describe a similar process. Only Hope does not match her *kippah* to her outfit. The others, as Becky explains, "pick it based on season, hour, and the rest of the ensemble." Ella was especially excited when her granddaughter selected a theme color for her bat mitzvah that matched the *tallis* that Ella wears. She smiles warmly and says, "I match my *kippah* to my outfit, but if I don't have one, I know I can always fall back on one of the ones from [my granddaughter's] bat mitzvah. They always match!"

Kippot wearing women also base their choices on function. Just as hair covering methods can be based on comfort (a *tichel* for exercise or sleep), ease (a snood while cleaning), or hat (for professional reasons), *kippot* are similarly selected. Carla slips off her *kippah* and gathers her short dirty blonde hair into a yellow snood that matches her dress and sunny personality. She explains, "Around the house, sometimes I like to wear a snood instead of a *kippah*. It stays on better when I'm taking care of the dogs or doing housework." Suzanne frequently bases her choice on the size of the *kippah*. She clarifies, "I have a small head. I need something that is going to stay on. Sometimes that means sacrificing fashion for function." Although she is always aware that not all colors compliment her fiery red hair and light complexion. Becky agrees, "When I'm teaching Hebrew school or doing stuff with the kids outside, I like to wear a fuller *kippah* that will stay on my head. But for fancy events, sometimes one of the wire ones looks nice. It's just not as practical, you know?"

Choosing appropriate head or hair covering based on function is often governed by social pressures largely from within the group. All of the women who wear some sort of covering identify certain social circumstances which influence their choices. In these instances the women engage in a triple consciousness,[17] in which they are aware of the careful balance they must maintain between their desires, the community's acceptance, and of gender norms which they face. That is to say, they base their actions on what their Jewish community expects, what they find spiritually or ritually enriching, and what it means to be a woman in a male-centered religious hierarchy.

Both groups of women tend to base their hair covering choices on social context: wearing particular types of coverings in order to either blend in or distinguish themselves from those around them. Their choices are influenced by the type of event. As Suzanne details, "A fun novelty *kippah* might be cute when I'm learning with someone, but I wouldn't wear it to a funeral or wedding!" Even though the women recognize that their head covering sets them apart as different from the other women around them, which is sometimes the intent of their actions, they are respectful of social norms. Becky carelessly twists her dark curls as she explains, "Just like I pick out what I'm going to wear based on where I am going, I do that with my *kippah*. I'm not going to wear a tie-died sundress to a funeral, just like I wouldn't wear a smiley face *kippah*."

Perhaps the most striking similarity in the ways in which the women interviewed describe their hair and head covering choices is in their perception of how the practices mark an externalization of their *Yiddishkeit*. Rachel, who looks the perfect combination of polished and carefree in her summer dress and sandals, explains, "I like that it makes me feel like I am completing my Jewish external look." Suzanne agrees, saying, "[It shows] that I'm making a conscious choice to show my Judaism on the outside."

This externalization seems to be especially important for women who have converted to Judaism. Both Orthodox and nonorthodox converts feel a sense of importance when conveying their Judaism. By covering their heads or hair, they mark this change and commitment not only to themselves, but also to their congregation and the local community. Beth, who converted to Reform Judaism, connects the two groups of women, explaining, "I think covering should be emphasized today. I think it is a part of our culture. I would like to see more women wear *kippot*. I see it as part of being Jewish. I actually admire Orthodox women who [cover their hair] with such intention, deliberation."

Underscored in Beth's statement of the similarity between head and hair covering is an understanding of the two as distinct practices. How is hair covering different than head covering? There are four primary ways that it varies: it is a reappropriation of a male practice; it indicates spirituality rather than observance; it connotes religious authority; and many of the women do not cover their heads in non-Jewish contexts.

In addition to their rhetorical choice to refer to their covering choices as *kippot* and not *yarmulkes*, the women also are sensitive to how their reappropriation of this male practice is perceived. Hope is critical of what she considers "feminized *kippot*." She identifies these head coverings as those which are embroidered with flowers, made in "girly colors," or otherwise marked as distinctly feminine. She explains, "[My *kippot*] are the same as men. I only have one that is embroidered with flowers that a man wouldn't be comfortable wearing. That one was a gift. The rest of 'em are unisex." The other women expressed less opposition to feminine *kippot*. Still, they oppose the idea that women should wear a female version of a *kippah*. Suzanne explains,

"I don't *have* to wear a feminine head covering, just like I don't have to wear a dress. But if I think it is pretty, why shouldn't I feel pretty?" Indeed, just as men might choose to wear a *kippah* with their favorite sports team's logo, is it really wrong for a woman to wear a design that appeals to her?

The answer that the women feel most comfortable with is that they should be able to wear feminine *kippot* if it is a personal style choice. However, they have just as much right to wear "masculine" *kippot* if they so choose. Carla offers an anecdote that aptly describes this differentiation. She quips, "At my first synagogue, there was a big discussion—whether a female rabbi should dress like a man or wear dresses. Eventually, the compromise position was that a woman rabbi should wear a suit with a frilly blouse and a girly *kippah*. . . . It was the stupidest stuff, but it was important to [the congregation]. I wanted to scream, I'm trying to teach *Midrash* here—my makeup, my blouse, the length of my skirt, the height of my heels, the color of my *kippah*, that has nothing to do with it! Get a grip!"

Their understanding of head covering as an egalitarian Jewish practice has an underlying understanding of the evolution of the tradition. Although they are uncomfortable labeling hair covering as "old world," they struggle to negotiate it with their own beliefs. Hope explains, "I feel that women who cover their hair with [the Orthodox] intent, I feel they are being submissive. . . . It's not that I'm opposed to the act as much as I am the philosophy." Suzanne, whose daughter went through a period of hair covering, details her mother's reaction, saying, "I accepted it, but my mother's reaction, well, she just couldn't understand it. It bothered her that my daughter was doing things that she had worked so hard to evolve away from." Indeed, the progression that the women generally perceive is:

The women interviewed believe that their choice to cover their heads is explicitly egalitarian. They have a deeply entrenched belief that, as Jews, it is their right—perhaps even their duty—to cover their heads. In principle, this has nothing to do with gender. It is a Jewish question, not a gendered decision. However, in reality, gender is at the heart of their choice. By covering their heads, they assert, as Carla describes, "That we are women, Jewish women, who live just as Jewishly as men, and we have all of the same rights."

When speaking about head covering, the women refer to it as a ritual or, less commonly, a practice that is important to them. Yet, when questioned about their levels of observance, they typically did not include head covering with other markers of observance (for example, keeping a kosher kitchen or regular Sabbath service attendance). Instead, they classify head covering as a spiritual endeavor. That is to say, rather than serving as a marker of Jewish observance, for them, head covering serves as an indicator of Jewish spirituality.

Their focus on spirituality instead of observance is in line with their Jewish affiliation. The women all self-identify as Reform or Conservative, movements that are often less or differently ritually observant than Orthodoxy. Still, spirituality is not the same buzz word for Jews as it is for Christians. What do these women mean when they speak of spirituality? When the women refer to covering their heads as spiritually enriching, they allude to two things: either they feel that head covering is a marker of how seriously they take Judaism, or they see head covering as an indicator of religious authority.

Carla explains, "I'm covering my head because of my sense of spirituality and also because I want to be identified with the Jewish people." Beth, fiddling with the Star of David charm on her necklace, agrees, saying, "[Covering my head] shows how important my religion is to me. 'Cause I'm making a conscious choice to do that, especially in a Reform synagogue, where, you know, choice is the word. I think it shows how seriously I feel about being Jewish." Becky expands on this idea, noting, "There isn't really any other way for me to say to people, to show them, how seriously I take being a Jew. It's such a big deal to me that it changes me inside and out."

Leaning back on her sofa with her legs casually crossed, Ella speaks of a "spiritual path" which led her to cover her head. After losing her parents at a young age, she is uncertain as to which Jewish practices were important to her family. She based her Jewish observance on what she remembered her parents doing; this includes her Orthodox mother covering her hair at Sabbath services. She explains, "I just did what I remembered and what I felt comfortable with. I remembered that covering your hair was a sign of respect." After moving away from Orthodoxy and choosing to affiliate with Conservative and ultimately Reform synagogues, one might expect that Ella would have abandoned the practice. Rather, her choice to cover her head has evolved into a deeply meaningful part of her spiritual life. She clarifies, "I think, in general, people tend to hearken back to their parents when they do things. But I cover my head and wear a *tallis* much more because of my daughters. They started doing it, and I felt like I should respect them enough. They both are much more serious students of Judaism than I am, and I have learned from that. It is really something that is very meaningful for me." She concludes, "My hair covering says to me that I live deeply in my Judaism. You don't need to be Orthodox to live a deeply spiritual life. What I do, I've learned from my daughters, who live fully as Jews. It's sort of a strange mixture of my mother and my daughters put together in me. Somehow I'm that link between them."

The ritualization of wearing *kippot* has evolved into a more contemporary and egalitarian expression of religious commitment. Although the women do not speak of it in terms of observance, it is their way of differentiating themselves from other Jewish women. The importance of their spirituality and religious beliefs are manifested through their head coverings. Head covering also serves to indicate religious authority. Not only does it mark the individual woman's authority to live fully as a Jew regardless of her gender, it also indicates religious authority for clergy.

In terms of indicating personal religious agency, the choice to cover their heads is decidedly feminist. In doing so, they indicate to viewers and to themselves that they have all of the same religious rights—and by extension, ritual expectations—as Jewish men. Becky, speaking just as much with her hands as her voice, explains, "If Jewish women are truly equal to Jewish men, and they're supposed to cover their heads, why aren't we all either collectively covering or not covering? Oh yeah, look at that guy, he must be really Jewish. He has on a yarmulke. My *kippah* says, but why not look at her? She must be really Jewish, too!" She goes on to say, "If we're gonna be truly egalitarian, with women at the *bimah*, women leading services, you know, the whole shebang, why aren't women wearing *kippot*? I do it to show that I have the right—no—as a Jew, I have the *obligation* to do all of this stuff."

When asked what their views were about female clergy covering their heads, the women struggled with whether or not the practice should be mandated. All of them agreed that it was important, several felt it should be required, but most felt that it should be a choice. Beth explains, "I feel like clergy should be required to cover their heads. I want my rabbi with a *kippah*, whether it's a male or a female. It indicates a dedication to Judaism. I know it's a choice, but I think that for clergy it's important." Hope agrees, adding, "They have accepted the authority and should show it."

Interestingly, the members of clergy interviewed were the ones who felt the most strongly about the importance of choice. Suzanne, with fire in her eyes to match her red hair, explains, "Female clergy should absolutely not be required to cover their heads! Male clergy aren't, so why should women?" Although she is not required to cover her head, Suzanne made the choice because, "It shows that I care, that I'm making a conscious choice to show my Judaism on the outside. And sure, I think it's a feminist statement, too, that I have the right to do it. That I have the right not only to wear the *kippah* but to do all of the other things in a synagogue that men do. I think it is a powerful statement. It communicates a lot."

Even if female clergy feel strongly that it is their choice to cover their heads, it seems that their congregants may actually desire that clergy take on the practice. Ella eloquently communicates the tension between desiring and mandating head covering. She explains, "I feel that female clergy should cover their heads, but I don't know if I think that. Clergy should be able to make determinations based on what they believe, especially since they've studied so much. But it would feel very strange for me to go to a service and see the person leading the service not wearing a *kippah*. It sort of feels disrespectful."

If wearing a *kippah* is not required of clergy and relatively few congregational women wear *kippot*, what types of reactions do these women experience from their congregation, families, and larger community? Much as Orthodox women cover their hair as a means of establishing boundaries within their community, *kippot* function as a separation mechanism for these women. This is demonstrated through the othering that occurs both within the synagogue and in the local community.

When asked about reactions to their choice to wear *kippot*, the women shared relatively similar stories in which they explained that although some friends and family were shocked, they anticipated this response, and it did not discourage them. For example, Hope saddens as she tells, "My aunt was mortified by my choice. She would never dream of doing it. And the women at my synagogue, a number of them made it clear that they didn't share my belief. They stared, made faces, you know." Ella describes that she was actually approached and told to go to another synagogue but that now, "They just deal with it. They've gotten used to me."

With such negative reactions, the women's continued wearing of *kippot* indicates how strongly they feel about the practice. If they were not so fully committed to covering their heads, surely social pressure would have caused them to abandon head covering. Yet, in the synagogue at least, it is an important way to establish social boundaries and demonstrate their *Yiddishkeit* and commitment to Judaism. *Kippot,* with their prominent placement on the head, strongly state that the women are committed to egalitarian religious practice. Their *kippot* say, as Becky describes, "We have the right to wear *kippot*. We are Jews. Not just female Jews. We are *Jews.*"

If *kippot* communicate so much within the synagogue, why do so few of the women wear them during their daily life? And if they do, what types of reactions do they receive? Very few Jewish women wear head coverings outside of Jewish contexts.

Although she does not wear a head covering on a daily basis, Suzanne describes her daughter's experience, saying, "[My daughter] decided she wanted to start wearing a *kippah* all the time. She wanted to be a rabbi. There were only three or four other Jewish kids in her school, and she had to get permission from the school and explained her choice to everybody. She was a bold teenager. She was brave! She only wore it for a few months, maybe just to prove that she could. It was a big statement! I was proud of her, both when she started and when she stopped. She made those decisions for herself."

Ella's daughter also covers her head daily. She tells of her daughter's struggle, saying, "My daughter recently spent a year in Jerusalem. She got such terrible looks and comments from others for wearing a *kippah* in public that she started wearing a hat instead. It's sort of ironic that the one place she couldn't feel comfortable wearing a *kippah* was in Israel! But in the US, there are fewer Jews, and most non-Jews just don't care."

Carla, who always wears a head covering, remarks, "I know it makes me a little bit weird, so I get some reaction." She goes on to explain that even though many women do not cover their heads, most Jewish men also appear bareheaded when outside of the synagogue. Still, she feels that like Jewish men who choose to consistently wear a yarmulke, she has made the choice to express her "street *Yiddishkeit*" to the larger community.

How the local community interprets Jewish female head covering, however, is an entirely different issue. Carla details, "Everyone around here wears some kind of head covering, the women at least. So people generally just assume I'm Mennonite." Beth, who covers her head all of *Shabbat* and has a strong desire to cover her head daily, admits, "It's really living here that keeps me from wearing [a *kippah*] all the time. If I lived somewhere else, I would probably start wearing it every day. 'Round here, I don't want to be mistaken as a Mennonite." Becky agrees, noting, "These Mennonite ladies smile at me and are all 'Hey Sister!' but I'm like, woah, wrong kind of sister! They have no idea!"

Although the women feel that their *kippot* represent their religious commitment and spirituality, the coverings are a misinterpreted marker in the localized context. Their *kippot* are a statement of agency, feminism, and their right as women to live fully as Jews. However, they are interpreted by the local community as a sign of female Christian submission. The contrast between the two is difficult to negotiate. Becky shrugs, "If it were easy, everyone would do it, right? So, even if they don't get it, I'm not going to give up." Carla agrees, "I don't have to lecture everyone about it and why I do it. Usually they just accept it is who I am as a person. But hey, at least around here, people don't stare at you as much as somewhere else. Sometimes, I'm glad for that. It lets me just do my own thing."

ACTIVE REINTERPRETATION AND RECONSTRUCTION OF RITUAL AND PRACTICE

Each time a woman puts on a *kippah*, she makes a statement to herself, to those in her congregation, and, at times, to those in the greater community. She says, "This is who I am—a Jewish female. This is my right as a Jew, regardless of my gender." Even if her actions are met with resistance or are misinterpreted by the larger community, her choice to cover her head is a statement of unapologetic egalitarianism.

Embedded in the choice of women to wear *kippot* is an underlying recognition that customs and rituals do not need to be Old World or patriarchal.

Rather, women have the power to transform ritual and practice and render it fulfilling, spiritually enriching, and egalitarian. That is to say, through their active engagement with traditional practice, contemporary Jewish women are able to reinterpret and reconstruct traditional behavior and belief to have it meet their needs and sensibilities.

Jewish feminists have paved the way for women to participate in synagogue life and have even concentrated on female affirming rituals like the celebration of *Rosh Chodesh* (the new Jewish month). Included in this, albeit on the periphery, has been religious dress. Contemporary nonorthodoxy Jewry generally has moved away from religious garb. Feminists have viewed the abandonment of hair covering and *tsnius* (modest) clothing as liberating. However, as the women interviewed in this chapter demonstrate, traditional attire is not necessarily oppressive. It is the intent with which it is worn. Women who cover their heads take a practice that is both traditional and male and prove that it is not a relic of the past. Rather, through their reappropriation and reinterpretation, head covering can be both ritually and spiritually fulfilling for contemporary Jewish women.

Their interest in and commitment to covering their heads demonstrates an active female engagement with tradition. Rather than abandoning tradition because of patriarchal undertones or the exclusion of women, they have chosen to embrace traditional behavior and modernize it. This forward thinking attitude demonstrates that Jewish women are claiming agency over their bodies as well as their spiritual life. They seek to externalize their internal beliefs, as well as claim their place within both the synagogue and the larger Jewish community.

Moving forward, the women have the hope that their actions will help to inspire other Jewish women, particularly young girls, to take control of their religious lives. Hope explains, "I feel it's my responsibility. It models behavior for girls and young women, to see what it means to be a Jewish woman." Carla agrees, saying, "My *kippah* tells girls, you can do this, too. And by doing [traditionally male rituals and practices], I hope to make the way easier for them to do it all, to feel like they can do it, that they have the right to do it, that they can decide what is spiritually enriching for them, regardless of their genitalia."

It is not that the women believe that all Jewish women have to uphold the same practices. Instead, their actions call for a careful evaluation of religious belief and application. They recognize the danger of stagnancy and support the continued evolution of Judaism. They understand Jewish women who choose not to cover their heads, but their concern is women who do not evaluate and consider their choices. Complacency, in this mindset, is far more dangerous than considerate traditionalism.

In a society where the trend is to privatize faith, by wearing *kippot*, these women make a strong public statement of their faith and beliefs. Their spirituality and commitment to Judaism is manifested externally, showing those around them that they are unapologetically Jewish. Perhaps even more importantly, their choice to cover their heads demands the right to practice traditions that had historically excluded them. Straightening the clip holding her *kippah* to her hair, Suzanne concludes, "Every once in a while someone will say, aren't *yarmulkes* for men? And I'll say, well, traditionally they're required for men, but there is nothing that says a woman can't [wear one]. So we do, because we can."

NOTES

1. Examples include, but certainly are not limited to: Shabbat 156b; Kiddushin 31a; Mishneh Torah, Ahavah, Hilkhot Tefilah 5:5; Shulchan Arukh, Orach Chayim 2:6

2. Shabbat 156b.

3. Eli Davis and Elise Davis, *Hats and Caps of the Jews* (Jerusalem: Masada, 1983), 17.

4. Davis and Davis, *Hats and Caps*, 17–19.

5. Davis and Davis, *Hats and Caps*, 318.

6. Jonathan D. Sarna, *American Judaism: A History* (New Haven: Yale University Press, 2005), 159.

7. Cyrus Adler, *American Jewish Yearbook: September 25, 1900 to September 13, 1901* (Philadelphia: Jewish Publication Society of America, 1901), 500.

8. Sarna, *American Judaism*, 161.

9. Davis and Davis, *Hats and Caps*, 160.

10. Suzanne Baizerman, "The Jewish *Kippah sruga* and the Social Construction of Gender in Israel," In *Dress and Gender: Making and Meaning*, ed. Ruth Barnes and Joanne B. Eicher (New York: Breg Publishers, 1992), 92–105.

11. Judith Plaskow, "Jewish Feminist Thought," in *History of Jewish Philosophy*, ed. Daniel H. Frank and Oliver Leaman (New York, Routledge, 1997), 885–95.

12. See Sylvia Barack Fishman, *A Breath of Life: Feminism in the American Jewish Community* (Waltham, MA; Brandeis University Press, 1995); Judith Plaskow, *Standing Again at Sinai: Judaism from a Feminist Perspective* (New York: Harper, 1991); Dayna Ruttenberg, ed. *Yentl's Revenge: The Next Wave of Jewish Feminism* (New York: Seal Press, 2001). Jewish feminism is forced to grapple with both historic and contemporary concerns. That is to say, in keeping with Jewish thought, Jewish feminism is mindful of the Torah and the legacy of rules for living that were established by the male writers of the Talmud. However, at the same time, they engage with contemporary feminist thought and attempt to apply it to a religious worldview that is steeped in patriarchy. I contend that Jewish feminism does not become unprogressive if it affirms that some Jewish women feel themselves most valued and validated when in traditional contexts. Instead, the great diversity of belief is representative of the importance and empowerment of determining one's own self-identity. The lifestyle of Orthodox women may be uncomfortable for progressive feminists, but their traditionalism is a valid, conscious, and pro-woman lifestyle choice. Just as Jewish feminists believe in agency and the power of self-identity, Orthodox women who have made the conscious and gender affirming choice to cover their hair have made a decision parallel to Jewish women who choose to cover their heads.

13. The difference in terminology between cantor and cantorial soloist stems from level of training. A cantor has completed a graduate degree and is invested (similar to rabbinic ordination). A cantorial soloist, on the other hand, has not completed a graduate degree and does not have all of the same training or authority as a cantor, despite performing many of the same liturgical functions.

14. It is possible to make the argument for the hair/head covering distinction for certain Plain Christian groups. However, in both cases the coverings' purpose is linked to the actual covering of hair, which is considered a woman's glory. There are some non-Plain Brethren and

Mennonite women who wear coverings at religious services, particularly communion, love-feast, and foot washing. Their choice to do so stems from a traditional understanding of the practice. Where they differ from Jewish women is that they have borrowed this practice from other women. That is to say, they are more similar to the women in chapter four who cover their hair as part of minhag. The Jewish women who cover their heads, however, have taken the practice from men to replace traditional female hair covering.

15. The women, like many American Jews, are inconsistent with how they pluralize Hebrew and Yiddish. For example, *kippot* was sometimes rendered *kippas*. Likewise, *tallisim* became *tallises*.

16. For some of the women, there is likely an underlying tension that feminism might be equated with a lesbian identity, hence causing them to shirk association with the word.

17. See W. E. B. DuBois, *The Souls of Black Folk* (New York: Gramercy Books, 1994). DuBois considers the idea of multiple consciousnesses, explaining what he observes as a double consciousness among African Americans.

Chapter Seven

The Long and Short of It

A Psychoreligious Interpretation of Hair Covering

As a child, aside from reading, my favorite form of entertainment was watching musicals that my mother had dutifully recorded from the classic movie channel onto VHS tapes. I suspect that I may have been the only child in suburban Philadelphia during the 1980s who thought a fun afternoon included singing or belting out a tune along with Judy Garland, Gene Kelly, Julie Andrews, and, most importantly, Barbra Streisand.

Recently I took a rare sick day to nurse a head cold. Unable to muster the motivation or strength to read or write during my day off, I indulged my inner child with a day of Streisand musicals. After working my way through *Funny Girl* and *Hello Dolly!*, two of my personal favorites, I remembered *Yentl*. This 1983 movie adaptation of the beloved story penned by Isaac Bashevis Singer titled, "Yentl the Yeshiva Boy" tells the story of a young woman desperate to study Talmud. After her father's death, she is alone in the world and decides to attempt to study at a *yeshiva* by pretending to be a man. The movie depicts Yentl slowly and deliberately cutting her hair short. Her transformation from woman to man is marked through the altering of her hairstyle.

Pausing the movie, I rushed to find my collection of Singer's short stories. Was this strictly theatrical or had Singer also realized that hair had such transformative powers? Sure enough, there in his story, Singer wrote:

> There was no doubt about it. Yentl was unlike any of the girls in Yaner—tall, thin, bony, with small breasts and narrow hips. On Sabbath afternoons, when her father slept, she would dress up in his trousers, his fringed garment, his silk coat, his skullcap, his velvet hat, and study her reflection in the mirror. She looked like a dark, handsome young man. There was even a slight down on her

117

upper lip. Only her thick braids showed her womanhood—and if it came to
that, hair could always be shorn. [1]

The rest of my sick day was a blur. I reread the story and finished watching
the movie, but I could not shake the nagging questions that it brought into my
mind. Was Yentl's choice to cut her hair a conscious or a subconscious
reaction to her change in self-identity and presentation? Is it possible that it
could be both? And if her choice existed both within and outside of her
awareness, what did it mean for the women that I studied? The only thing
about which I was certain was that an old Streisand movie had moved from
fond childhood memory to incredibly relevant in my adult life.

CREATING A PSYCHORELIGIOUS APPROACH

In this chapter I identify a psychoreligious approach, based on Erich
Fromm's *Psychoanalysis and Religion*. I use Fromm's consideration of the
subconscious motivations of human needs to process and interpret the material gathered through ethnographic observations, interviews, and symbolic
inventory. Ultimately I argue that Orthodox women and their choices are
responsible for the continuation of American Orthodoxy, which is especially
true in small communities.

Erich Fromm, a famous German-American psychoanalyst, is perhaps best
known for his work in political psychology questioning the cognition of
freedom. [2] However, although less recognized, his work in the psychology of
religion is pivotal for those interested in psychoanalytically investigating
religion. Religion has traditionally been left out of psychoanalytic approaches, as it is not considered a matter of individual development and is
subject to the bias of the analyst (such as Freud's analysis of Judaism as a
Jew). Understanding his cultural psychoanalytic approach will frame my
psychoreligious analysis of women who cover their hair.

Born to Orthodox parents and descended from a long line of Talmudic
scholars and rabbis, [3] it is no wonder that Fromm was reticent to completely
dismiss religion. As a student of the Talmud, Fromm believed that psychoanalysis and religion could harmoniously coexist and enrich one another. [4]
His investigation of this idea began with his dissertation, *Das jüdische Gesetz: Ein Beitrag zur Soziologie des Diaspora-Judentums (Jewish Law: A
Sociological Study of Jewish Diaspora)*, which he completed in 1922. In this
work, he considers how *halakha* functions to maintain a continued Jewish
cultural affiliation despite the tensions of living as a diasporic people. Although he did not yet have the tools of psychoanalysis at his disposal, he
spoke of the "Jewish social body" being held together by "social cement,"
which he saw as an adherence to *halakha* despite conflicting social norms
within the host culture. This daily adherence to Jewish ritual fostered solidar-

ity, community identification, and helped to negotiate the tensions of living in Diaspora.[5]

As Fromm's psychoanalytic theory developed, he identified several basic subconscious human needs, including the need to feel rooted (or a sense of belonging), the desire to have a sense of identity both as an individual and as part of a group, and, by extension, the need to feel unity with others.[6] All of these identities manifest in religious desire, commitment, and belief. Unlike Freud, who sees religion as a coping mechanism and God as a father figure replacement,[7] Fromm understands religion as an avenue to "becoming aware of life and of one's own existence, and of the puzzling problem of one's relatedness to the world."[8] Although Fromm considers Jung to be more accepting of religion, he fears that Jung "elevates the unconscious to a religious phenomenon."[9] Fromm's approach to religion is attuned to the "ultimate concern with the meaning of life, with the self-realization of man, with the fulfillment of the task which life sets us" and is "an attitude of oneness not only in oneself, not only with one's fellow men, but with all life and, beyond that, with the universe."[10] In other words, Fromm does not consider religious belief neurotic or a sign of weakness. Rather, he sees it as a motivation to connect with others in a meaningful way which meets the basic subconscious desire to live a fulfilled life.

If we consider some of the basic human needs that Fromm identifies (rootedness, identity as an individual and group, and feeling unity with others), the importance of religious ritual emerges. Ritual, particularly for a diasporic community, functions to create interconnectivity and community allegiance. However, psychoanalysts have traditionally considered ritual as a pathological expression of compulsion. There is, however, an important distinction to be made between compulsive/irrational ritual and rational ritual.

Hand washing is a clear example of this. Those who obsessively or compulsively wash their hands out of a fear for germs engage in an irrational ritual. They are governed by a compulsive need for cleanliness and fear what will happen to them if they fail to wash their hands properly, often enough, or in a certain way. This is, however, drastically different from ritualized religious hand washing. Orthodox Jews who engage in *netilat yadayim* (ritual hand washing, in Yiddish, *negel vasser*) uphold the practice as a rational ritual. Although they may feel guilt if they fail to wash their hands properly at prescribed times, they are not compulsively driven to engage in the ritual. Rather, it is an extension of their religious belief and identity. Their lives are not governed by ritual compulsion.

Another clear example of this is fasting. A woman with an eating disorder allows irrational fasting rituals to govern her life. She fears what will happen to her if she eats. Religious fasting holidays, on the other hand, are a practice rather than a compulsion. Those fasting feel an obligation or desire to abstain from eating, but it is an exercise in self-restraint in order to focus on spirituality rather than a fear-driven, compulsive eating ritual. In the end, the consumption of food is celebrated to mark the end of the fast. This approach is in line with Theodor Reik and the idea of functionalism. Reik and Fromm's understanding suggests that, rather than being bizarre, rituals and customs are intentionally framed to provide symbols and functions for a group, thereby confirming identity and values, effecting internal social solidarity and differences from other groups, and providing life passage. In this sense rituals are not a pathology but part of a social process. They are often tenuous because they rely on compliance and therefore are negotiated, and in the process reveal tensions and anxieties in a group's psychology.[11]

If we accept that there is a fundamental difference between rational and irrational rituals, and we accept that a rational ritual is, as Fromm explains, a "shared action expressive of common strivings rooted in common values,"[12] how do we negotiate religious ritual with psychoanalysis? First, we must accept that not all religious rituals will seem rational to us. Religious culture is diverse and what seems to be irrational to one person may be meaningful and rational for another. Second, we need to understand that religious ritual is a symbolic language that expresses belief through action.[13] Religious ritual employs a separate symbol set that outsiders may not always understand. Third, if we accept Fromm's theory that humans have a fundamental desire to feel connected with a community, religious ritual is a manifestation of that desire.

Therefore, ritual is both a conscious and subconscious expression. To identify ritual as strictly conscious negates the motivating factors for ritual that may exist outside of the awareness of the individual. However, to consider ritual strictly as a subconscious phenomenon ignores the cultural and sociological influences and pressures that an individual experiences. Rational religious ritual, then, operates on both a conscious and subconscious level.

These ideas taken together are the basis of my psychoreligious approach. This method considers religious belief, practice, and ritual to function on both the conscious and subconscious level. Religious practice which is, in this case, external manifestations of ritual and belief through hair and hair covering exists both within and outside of the awareness of the individuals. Degel Israel women's choices are influenced by the secular world, their religious community, self-agency, and subconscious needs. I identify functions of religious beliefs and practices and their effect on social relations and cultural viability. I relate these practices to the identity of the group, particularly in the conduct of everyday life outside of the "frame" of the congregation. I concentrate on evaluating the special role of hair covering and its function of negotiating religious identity in a small non-Jewish city, questioning why it has taken on special importance in this context.

HAIR COVERING AS A CONSCIOUS AND
SUBCONSCIOUS CHOICE

When discussing religious ritual, costuming and hair are generally excluded. In some ways, this is understandable. Unlike other ritualized behavior such as the washing of hands or fasting, clothing and hair do not perform formal or institutionalized religious function. However, as Solomon Poll notes, for Orthodox Jews, "Religion determines the characteristic form of most activities, so much so that even secular activities have come to acquire a religious meaning."[14] That is to say, costuming and hair, although not considered religious ritual by practitioners, are examples of ritualized behavior. Poll goes on to explain that "the main object of [Hasidic] existence is the perpetuation of *Yiddishkeit*, traditional religious Judaism," which is only achieved through particular convictions and behavior.[15] In other words, Poll asserts that in order for a countercultural religious community to survive, they must imbue all of their activities religiously, which Poll calls a "superordinate meaning system."[16] In doing so, the group establishes intra-community norms that help to negotiate the pressure to assimilate into the dominant culture.

Poll emphasizes the importance of ritual, which he sees as a way to consistently reidentify with the Orthodox community. He explains that rituals extend beyond those that are publically expressed to include rituals that occur privately throughout the day. In this case, ritual is both spiritual and performative, functioning to create both a sense of belonging for the individual as well as a control mechanism for the community.[17] In order for religious ritual to be so encompassing of daily life, Orthodox Jews, and in Poll's consideration, particularly Hasidim, must religiously identify secular actions and objects. Poll gives the example of heavy-gauge stockings, which might in other contexts be considered insignificant hosiery. However, for Hasidim these stockings are a religious symbol of group belonging, functioning as part of a costuming hierarchy that indicates levels of religious observance.[18] This idea can be extended to include hair covering practices as a form of performative and meaningful externalizations of religious belief and community identification.

If we accept that hair covering is performative and individualized, how does it relate to religious ritual? In order to evaluate this question, we will consider the three aspects of rational ritual identified as part of my psychoreligious approach: not all ritual will seem rational to us, religious ritual is a symbolic language that expresses belief through action, and religious ritual is a manifestation of community connectivity.

Those of us who are bareheaded may not understand the feelings experienced or motivations of those who cover their hair. Those who do cover their hair find it both spiritually and personally fulfilling. Hair and hair covering are used in a variety of ways across cultures. Although it may be unfamiliar or even undesirable for those outside of the culture, for Orthodox Jews, female hair covering is a ritualized practice deeply steeped in tradition. Likewise, going bareheaded also implies a symbolic practice, even though in the majority society it is not considered so. In larger American culture, bareheadedness is thought of as normative and therefore taken for granted. Yet to the religious it marks the "other" world about which one may have ambivalent feelings. In religious thought this relates to the idea of "two kingdoms"—evil or dangerous worldly and the righteous or obedient minority—as a worldview.

For some outsiders, hair covering is misunderstood to represent female submission. However, for the women who choose to cover their hair, they believe their hair covering practices demonstrate their commitment to Judaism. For these women, the choice is empowering. It marks female entry into the male-centered Judaic ritual system, a change in focus which the women embrace. Rather than indicating submission, hair covering for Orthodox women demonstrates power and religious responsibility.

Hair covering is also linked to religious ritual through the symbolic language with which it communicates belief. These beliefs are translated into action—in this case, the covering of hair—which convey messages to both the wearer and the viewer. [19] The symbolic set functions both on an individual and religious community level.

For individuals, hair functions as a manifestation of personal belief. As the women in chapter four described, their daily choice to cover their hair affirmed their spiritual commitment. They use hair coverings to symbolically convey their various levels of observance. They vary their hair covering based on context, comfort, and personal style. Each morning when they put on their hair covering, Orthodox women make a ritualized choice to externally mark themselves, reaffirming their constant commitment to living an Orthodox lifestyle.

Women also make a choice to identify with a particular strain of Orthodoxy when they select their method of hair covering. This process also functions on an individual as well as a community level. For the individual, it represents her allegiance to the group, to their collective level of observance, and to raising her children in line with their shared belief system. As a community symbol, the choice to cover hair in the same way demonstrates community cohesion. For those familiar with Orthodoxy, certain hair covering styles alert the viewer of community identification. Conservative hair covering typically indicates a higher level of religious observance.

Within the Orthodox community hair covering functions as an inclusionary marker. Much like high school social cliques have a certain "look" in the way that they dress, strains of Orthodoxy also have an external marking system. If a woman wants to identify with her community, her hair covering is the key symbol she uses to indicate her group allegiance. Similarly, if she wishes to change her identity or realign with another Orthodox community, she can symbolically alter her self-presentation through the use of her hair covering to represent this change.

This indication of community identification ties in to the idea of rational ritual functioning as a manifestation of community connectivity. A community defines itself with shared actions and beliefs. One of the clearest ways of doing this is through the externalization of ritual through clothing or hair.[20] This externalization is a public way of announcing affiliation with a particular community, as well as a private way of establishing a personal relationship with the group.

A shared sense of community identification is cultivated through common ritual. These moments of communal action are what maintain the group's collective identity. By enacting shared behavior, not only do members demonstrate their allegiance to Orthodoxy, but they also reinforce their own sense of belonging. This perception of rootedness is critical to the community's maintenance of both boundaries and membership. Ritual, in this case, regulates orthodox affiliation as well as establishes a sense of collective identity.[21]

If we accept that hair covering meets the three qualifiers for rational ritual, how does it function on the conscious and subconscious level for the women who cover their hair? In order to address this we will consider three of the basic needs which Fromm identifies: the need to feel rooted, the desire to have a sense of identity, and the need to feel unity.

Fromm considers the need to feel rooted as the subconscious desire to experience a sense of belonging, which surely also functions on a conscious level. In particular, an American context that tempers this study is the idea that American society is highly individualistic, putting into question one's need for social belonging. The women profiled in this study are consciously aware that some of their decisions foster this sense of belonging. For example, their choice to pay membership at Degel Israel is a literal statement of community membership. However, subconsciously they also desire a sense of rootedness. This is evidenced in two ways: in their desire to uphold tradition and in their desire to be taken seriously as Jews.

In an ever changing world where tradition is often discredited or considered "old world," Orthodox women are constantly bombarded with messages that threaten their adherence to traditional belief and ritual. However, the Orthodox social structure is based on traditional thought and the deferment of the individual to the community. Subconsciously the women desire affiliation with a community that affirms their lifestyle choices and belief in tradition. This counterculturalist desire manifests in the need to both feel separate from the larger secular world while at the same time feeling rooted and connected in their traditional lifestyle. It affirms the collective wisdom of the group. Just as their foremothers upheld traditional practices, contemporary Orthodox women find their roots in modeling their behavior and belief.

At the same time that they identify with past generations of Jewish women, Orthodox women also find their role in Judaism affirmed through hair covering. In a religion that is considered male-centered, hair covering accords women their own female ritual. Much of Jewish male ritual obligation is time-bound and daily (for example, laying *tefillin*, wearing *tzitzit*, or reciting the *Shema* in the morning and evening). Women, however, are generally exempt from time-bound *mitzvot* (commandments). Hair covering functions as a daily ritual that meets their needs to externally demonstrate their level of observance.

Much of Orthodox female ritual is private: for example, keeping a kosher kitchen or upholding sexual purity laws. Hair covering fills the subconscious need to externalize their sense of Jewish belonging. It marks them as observant Jews and serves as a daily reminder of their affiliation. It is their way of saying to others that they take being a Jew seriously and are committed to the Orthodox lifestyle. Although Orthodoxy may afford them few public ways of demonstrating this commitment, their desire to do so manifests in their use of hair covering over which they maintain control.

Fromm identifies another basic subconscious human need as the desire to have a sense of identity both as an individual and as part of a group. In the context of a modern society that opens identity to individual decisions rather than relying solely on tradition and in the process creates conflicts between parents and children, their desire centers religion as a prime identity. Hair covering meets this need in three ways: it establishes a tri-identity for the women, it validates separate gender roles, and it affirms womanhood.

Orthodox women must negotiate a complicated identity. During the work week, they largely live as assimilated American women. At the synagogue and other religious events, they must function as Orthodox women. Cognitively they must merge these two conflicting concepts of self together into a third identity: how they truly perceive themselves, free of the external pressures of American or Orthodox culture.

A way they negotiate this tri-identity is through hair covering. They vary their hair covering choices based on situation as well as personal preference. Outside of the Orthodox community, they may seek to blend in and appear fairly assimilated as an effort to alleviate some of the pressures they feel based on assumptions that the secular world makes about them. Within the Orthodox community, they identify with particular strains of Orthodoxy through their hair covering choices. Most importantly, however, is how their hair covering is an extension of their self-perception.

Orthodox women manipulate hair covering to demonstrate their self-perceived uniqueness. For example, they may accessorize a *tichel* with a broach or a headband, choose specific colors in which they feel most confident, or select hats that are quirky, whimsical, serious, or understated. Likewise, *sheitels* present the opportunity to change hair color and style. Much like women dye their hair to feel like a blonde bombshell or a fiery redhead, *sheitels* also allow Orthodox women to externalize perceived personality, whether that be Jewish, relate to attractiveness, or indicate expressions or levels of femininity. In this way, hair covering fulfills the desire to have a sense of individual identity, while at the same time allowing the wearer to conform to overall group expectations.

Orthodox women who cover their hair belong to a community that affirms separate gender roles. They are taught that women and men are fundamentally different, socially as well as biologically. They relate to social structure based on assigned gender roles to maintain separateness. This does not necessarily mean that they believe in inequality between the sexes; instead, gender plays an operative role in almost every aspect of their lives. From their religious obligations to their duties in the home, Orthodox women are taught that they have different expectations and responsibilities than men. Hair covering is a manifestation of this gendered difference.

As Orthodox women work to establish a sense of self-identity, a key element in their subconscious formation of the perception of self is of their separateness as women. They have culturally been taught that their gender sets them apart from men. As noted before, much of their religious obligations are private and not externalized. For them to feel like they manifest their religious affiliation, especially their identity as a Jewish *woman*, their one choice for externalization is hair covering.

Within Orthodox culture, there is no shame in recognizing gendered difference. The women embrace gendered difference as part of their religious worldview. They take pride in upholding rituals and practices that affirm the separation of the sexes. Whether it is wearing skirts rather than pants, visiting the *mikveh*, or taking responsibility for lighting Sabbath candles, Orthodox women understand these tasks to represent their Jewish femininity.

One of the greatest tasks entreated to Orthodox women is the creation and maintenance of a Jewish home. Beyond keeping a kosher kitchen, this means raising Jewish children who are taught to be religiously observant, to honor Judaism, and to uphold tradition. Mothers are implored to model behavior for their families, ensure that their children receive a proper Jewish education, and to create a home environment that is decidedly Orthodox. This type of household management is no small feat. However, the tasks which are conducted within the home are not visible to the public. Such work does not receive adequate recognition for its importance in maintaining the Orthodox social structure. This work, in fact, epitomizes what it means to be an Orthodox woman.

If Orthodox women accept their gendered difference, hair covering is the way through which they reclaim their femininity. It is an external manifestation of Judaism that is uniquely female. Hair covering demonstrates their commitment to gendered difference, while at the same time empowering them to make a statement about their own personal dedication to leading an observant life. It demonstrates to secular society that they accept their role as gendered bodies within Judaism. At the same time, it demonstrates to the Orthodox community that they have agency over their bodies and self-presentation. They are claiming their bodies as uniquely female and take pride in their femininity as part of their perceived gendered difference.

Although male Orthodox dress is often distinctive (caftans, knee socks, *shtreimels*, *yarmulkes*, and *payot*, for example), the female Orthodox version appears to be appropriate to person assimilated to the majority culture. Although women adhere to modest dressing principles, they purchase their clothing in secular department stores. Their clothing may be less revealing than most other American women, but it does not necessarily mark them as Orthodox. Hair covering, on the other hand, sets them apart from the secular world and aligns them with other Orthodox women. In this way it is an affirmation of their womanhood.

When outside of the Orthodox community, the women are bombarded by what it means to be "an American woman." Advertisements, magazines, television, movies, and even the women on the street communicate volumes with their bodies. Scantily clad images of models in lingerie tell women that sex sells and that it is through the display the body that one marks herself as feminine. However, Orthodox women receive a conflicting message from their religious community. They are taught that the body can produce lustful and distracting thoughts for men. Their "womanhood," therefore, should be concealed and saved for their husbands' eyes. How are they to feel affirmed in their womanhood if secular culture is telling them to reveal their bodies and their Orthodox culture is telling them to conceal themselves?

Despite the hypersexualization of American culture, Orthodox women find empowerment in concealing their bodies and hair. Rather than accepting the secular influence of revealing themselves in order to feel attractive, they express beauty in other ways. The goal of modest dressing and hair covering is not to appear dowdy. Instead, Orthodox women generally express that they feel *more* feminine when covering their bodies and hair. They attribute this to the empowerment of the desexualization of their bodies.[22]

Even nonorthodox women can understand the objectification that American women feel in terms of how their bodies are perceived. Just as female politicians and business professionals wear power suits to demonstrate their authority, Orthodox women see hair covering as a method of desexualizing themselves in order to gain power. With the focus off of their bodies and hair, they believe that they are seen for who they truly are. They are valued for their thoughts, insights, and contributions, rather than for their sex appeal. Feminists might critique hair covering as oppressive to women, but for Orthodox women, hair covering represents a way to present the true self that is not seen through the male sexualized lens.

Likewise, hair covering affirms womanhood through the link to gendered difference. Orthodox women see it is part of what it means to be a woman, saying things like, "My hair is my glory" or "I love how my hair makes me feel like a girl!" Their hair and body are alluring to men, and by concealing them, they accept not only their appeal but also their right to be treated as individuals rather than sex objects. They can choose when and how they wish to be sexually appealing. They reserve their hair for their husbands' eyes and touch and thereby gain sexual agency.

Similarly, Orthodox women feel affirmed through their feminine self-presentation. For them, wearing dresses, covering their hair, putting on makeup, and accessorizing their outfits is an enjoyable part of being a woman. As one woman described, "You know that old song, "I Enjoy Being a Girl?" Well, I really do! I love to get all dolled up. I love the way it makes me feel about myself!" Femininity is not something which is frowned upon within Orthodoxy, and women take pride in feeling womanly. In this case, hair covering demonstrates that a married female is still a woman: she still has the potential to be attractive to other men, even after giving birth to multiple children. She is still an object of desire and a sexual being, an idea which she embraces when she chooses to cover her hair.

The final basic subconscious need which we will consider is what Fromm as the desire to feel unity. For Orthodox women, hair covering is used to meet this need through the claiming of ritual, a reaction to feminism, and desire to maintain a separateness within a defined and connected community.

As discussed by Poll, one of the key ways with which a community maintains its sense of distinctness is through the use of ritual. For Orthodox women, hair covering is a subconscious claiming of ritual in order to maintain continued affiliation with the movement. They are aware of outsiders' perception of the patriarchal leanings of Orthodoxy. Moreover, Orthodox women are cognizant of feminism and its impact on contemporary American culture. Still, they are not ready to abandon traditional Judaism.

Their way of negotiating this difficulty is through the reclaiming of ritual, subverting something that could be seen as oppressive for women and rendering it empowering. After World War II, many Orthodox women abandoned hair covering. As seen in the stories of the women interviewed, most of them do not recall their mothers or grandmothers covering their hair. However, they have made the choice for themselves and their daughters are largely following in their footsteps. Their choice to cover their hair represents a conscious choice to engage in Jewish practice and a subconscious choice to claim and reinterpret ritual to accommodate the pressures that they feel from the secular world.

Moving away from Fromm's assumptions, in this way, their choice to cover their hair is also a subconscious reaction to feminism. Orthodox women are reticent to label themselves as feminists. However, their hair covering choices can be construed as profoundly feminist. Unknowingly they speak of their choice to cover their hair using feminist rhetoric: speaking of agency, empowerment, affirmation of womanhood, and of self-identity. Surely this approach to hair covering was not always the case for Orthodox women. Their great-grandmothers accepted hair covering as an obligation rather than an option. Contemporary Orthodox women consider hair covering their individual choice.

Without knowingly engaging with feminist ideas, Orthodox women are constantly confronted with America's evolving sense of what it means to be an empowered American woman. Having internalized the cultural norm that women should have agency over their bodies and lifestyle choices, Orthodox women have applied feminist theory to their own religious practices. This concept of choice has unintentionally cemented them as a cohesive unit. They constitute a group who has chosen to uphold tradition as a means of affirming their place within Judaism and their religious obligations and rights as traditional women.

An extension of this unity within tradition is their shared desire to maintain a feeling of separateness, while still fostering a sense of shared community and connectivity. Unlike other sectarian groups like the Amish or Hutterites, who have worked to remove themselves from the secular world, Orthodox Jews live very much as a part of secular America. Still, they understand themselves to be fundamentally different from typical Americans. This separateness creates a sense of unity in terms of their identification with their defined community, as well as in their united front with which they approach the secular world.

Female hair covering clearly articulates the coexistence of separateness and assimilation. In secular contexts, Orthodox women identify themselves as markedly different with their hair covering. However, it does not prohibit them from functioning in the secular world. Likewise, Jewish hair covering does not carry the same stigmas as some other forms of religious dress, for example the *burqua* or *niqab*. Similarly, though, Jewish female hair covering serves as a constant reminder to Orthodox women that they are not like their secular peers and Anabaptist cognates.[23] In most ways they may be fully assimilated into American culture, but there is still a fundamental difference—one that is articulated through their hair covering choice. That is to say, although Orthodox women may be culturally fluent in the secular world, they create and maintain a boundary between themselves and American culture through their choice to cover their hair.

Just as hair covering marks them as separate and different from the secular world, it also maintains a sense of communal unity within Orthodoxy.

Women who choose to cover their hair mark themselves as dually allegiant. The general choice to cover the hair indicates that a woman is observant and self-identifies as Orthodox. The deeper symbolism comes from how she chooses to cover her hair. Her choice of hair covering indicates with which strain of Orthodoxy she affiliates or identifies. In this case, it is an externalization of a cognitive symbol in order to effect unity.

HAIR COVERING AND THE FUTURE OF
AMERICAN ORTHODOXY

Clearly hair covering has a profound impact on Orthodox women—both on conscious and subconscious levels. What is its significance, though, beyond functioning as part of ritualized behavior or religious costuming? The importance of hair covering rests in the outward demonstration of female dedication to Orthodoxy and how this commitment ensures the survival of Orthodox Judaism for future generations. This is demonstrated through antiassimilationism and the uplifting of female ritual. The irony, of course, is that while this practice is an outward demonstration, it may not be perceived correctly in normative society. This raises the question of for whom the demonstration is—the self, popular culture, or other Orthodox or nonorthodox Jews.

In order for any countercultural movement to survive, the group must make a concentrated effort to protect its members from assimilating into the dominant culture. In most cases, this is done through minimizing interaction with the secular world. However, Orthodox Jews engage with American culture and are generally socially fluent in both American and Orthodox culture. For Orthodox Jews, it is not a conflict of interest to identify and engage with American culture. It is, however, an issue if the secular cultural norms come in conflict with religious obligations.

There are several ways in which Orthodox Jews remind themselves of their difference from the secular world. One of the clearest examples is *kashrut*, which serves as a constant reminder of their countercultural lifestyle choices. Hair covering, however, functions in a special way for Orthodox women. It is both a public and private announcement of their affiliation. Publically it marks them as different from their secular colleagues or friends. With its prominent placement on the head, it is an expression of their religious beliefs. Privately, though, it is also a meaningful practice. Hair covering is more than just ritual; it is a deeply spiritual practice that some Orthodox women see as crucial to expressing their religious belief. Even if the larger secular society does not always understand the messages that hair covering communicates, the practice is richly symbolic and meaningful for the women who engage in the practice.

Orthodox women who cover their hair demonstrate for future generations of Orthodoxy that there is a way to be publically and privately observant. Likewise, the ways in which they imbue daily practices, like hair covering, with spirituality allows them to live religiously within the secular world. Although they are antiassimilation, they are not closed off to the influences of American secular culture. It is this attitude that has allowed Orthodoxy to continue to grow and retain membership. Indeed, it is largely Orthodox women who decide just how secularly fluent their family will be. They are generally responsible for the educational choices of their children, for the consumer items which enter the home, and for the selection of clothing, entertainment, and books for their family. These decisions communicate volumes, as does a mother's choice to cover her hair. In doing so, she shows her children that she is able to function fully in the secular world without assimilating into the dominant culture. This lesson, coupled with her modeled behavior, profoundly influences her family.

There has been a renewed interest in hair covering in the last generation of Orthodox women. This could be interpreted to indicate a response to the increased pressure to assimilate, but it is even more likely that this new interest in covering hair is an extension of an increased desire to uplift and reinterpret female ritual. As Orthodox women engage in a careful balancing act where they must constantly negotiate secular and religious culture, they are influenced by pressures from both sides. As an extension of this, they are also affected by secular culture's consideration of what it means to be valued as a woman.

The women in this study are well aware of what feminism has meant in society and how this has at times conflicted with their religious social structure. They are not, however, entirely removed from these changes. Unlike previous generations when women were expected to stay in the home, contemporary American women have different expectations of self-autonomy and choice than their foremothers. Orthodox women have been influenced by this as well. As has been shown with the women profiled in this study, they are highly educated and are employed in a variety of fields. They have moved, for the most part, outside of the home. Their roles in the secular community have been revalued. Why should they not also reevaluate their roles in the Orthodox religious community?

The way in which Orthodox women have negotiated the tensions of feminism and traditional belief is in the reconceptualization of female ritual. In doing so, they emphasize their belief in gendered difference while stressing the importance of the role of women. When considering Jewish ritual and *halakha*, there are a limited number of uniquely female practices which Orthodox women have at their disposal. Sexual purity laws, the baking of *challah*, and the lighting of Sabbath candles are all uniquely female *mitzvot*. None of these rituals is regulated by men. However, all of these practices are private and associated with the home. Hair covering, in contrast, is public and linked to the individual. It enables Orthodox women to demonstrate their importance in both the home and the community, privately and publically.

Hair covering also enables Orthodox women to negotiate the idea of self-agency and choice with traditional values. They make a daily effort to cover their hair, which demonstrates their spiritual agency. In this way, they model for their daughters that Orthodox femininity does not equate to passivity. They are actively engaged in their religious lives, and this feeling of agency translates into empowerment. Without this feeling, it is likely that Orthodox women would feel greater pressure to succumb to assimilation. By covering their hair, the women establish a thoughtful boundary between themselves and the secular world. At the same time, they demonstrate the remarkable adaptability of Orthodox ritual to both stay true to tradition while still evolving to meet the needs of contemporary Orthodoxy.

Taken together, a clear picture begins to emerge that Orthodox women faced with ambivalence about their position in normative and religious cultures in a small city setting such as Lancaster often find their roles submerged or overlooked. However, they are largely responsible for the continuation of American Orthodoxy in their community. They create and maintain Orthodox homes; they are responsible for the Jewish education of their children; maintaining a kosher kitchen is their task; they volunteer and keep the local Jewish community running. At the same time, they typically work full time jobs, have pursued educational opportunities, and retain social connections both in the secular and religious community. All of these responsibilities are even more pronounced in a small-town Orthodox synagogue. In fact, the female workload is significantly higher in small communities. Not only are there fewer women between which to divide the work, but there are additional hurdles, like commuting long distances to purchase kosher foodstuffs, that further complicate their lives.

The choice to cover one's hair is a profound decision. It represents a steadfast commitment to Orthodoxy, demonstrates a high level of private religious observance, and, at the same time, is also spiritually meaningful for the woman. Moreover, especially in small communities, hair covering helps to negotiate the tension of living a countercultural lifestyle. It sets the women apart from the secular world while still allowing them to function within it. It also works as a coping mechanism that allows women to engage in self-expression at the same time as identifying as part of a greater religious whole.

As we head into the future, I suspect that hair covering will continue to experience ebbs and flows in popularity. However, since the practice has been reinterpreted and revalued as a uniquely female ritual, I believe that Orthodox women will continue to have an increased interest in covering their hair. Surrounded by a hypersexualized world which they constantly must negotiate with their religious beliefs, the practice of hair covering revalues a woman's body. It gives her agency over her presentation of self, as well as allowing her to claim her place within the patriarchal system of Orthodoxy. It affirms her belief in tradition, marking the roots from which she has grown and linking her to past generations of Jewish women. It also affirms her relationship to her Orthodox sisters and the religious community's collective wisdom to which she defers. Finally, hair covering indicates to future generations the importance that religious observance and commitment to tradition. In this way, she establishes herself as part of the roots for future generations of Orthodox Jews. She says to the world, as Debbie articulated, "Yes, I am an observant Jew. I'm proud of it. I don't really care what you think. Here it is!"

CONCLUSION: WEAVING THE FABRIC OF AMERICAN JUDAISM

In this study I have brought the voices of Orthodox women into the conversation of the issues facing contemporary American Orthodoxy. I have been especially attuned to the narratives of observant Jews living in small communities, recognizing that they are not heard or collected by scholars working with concentrated populations of pietistic Jews in metropolitan areas. Using hair study to understand the identities of these women, I have probed questions of how their context, location, gender role, and religious belief influence their approach to tradition and ritual. When looked at collectively, I have highlighted several key points.

First, and in my opinion most importantly, it is the women's situated context in a small community that has informed their cultural practices. The tensions that they face because of their location in a nonmetropolitan area surface in their use of hair covering practices. The different methods and forms of hair covering provide the structure that would typically come from the formal institution of the synagogue. However, in the nonmetropolitan context where the synagogue does not exert the same social control, strictures are self-imposed and regulated by the women.

Second, it is the women's interest and desire to have a feminized Jewish ritual that has made hair covering particularly appealing. Although Orthodox women are vocally against assimilation within dominant American society, they are not closed off to the influences of American secular culture. They have been affected by and are aware of feminism [24] and have willingly accepted many changes: for example, working outside of the home and embracing higher education. [25] Although Orthodox women have not embraced all of Jewish egalitarianism, such as the ordination of female clergy or the inclusion of women when counting *minyan*, they are aware of these changes. [26] In a parallel movement, they have demonstrated an increased desire to consider what it means to be both a woman and an Orthodox Jew. [27]

As I have discussed, much of what is uniquely feminine in Jewish ritual (lighting candles, *challah*, sexual purity laws) is private as are many of their other religious obligations (keeping a kosher kitchen, raising a Jewish family). However, hair covering represents a distinctly female and woman-controlled externalization of spirituality and religious commitment.

Third, the women profiled in this study use symbolic inventories with multilayered symbols. They engage in self-presentation that is encoded with different meanings for the women as well as to various audiences. Rather than blindly following tradition, the women creatively and strategically craft their ethnic religious self-presentation.[28] Other studies have marginalized their experiences or simplified them in such a way that renders their experiences secondary. Although it is true that male rabbinical leadership and the lack of Jewish affiliation and abundance of Jewish assimilation are key obstacles facing contemporary Jewry, these are not the only issues that confront American Jews. I contend that material and bodily practices are critical as tools of feminine empowerment. Likewise, they are practices which express identity and have been overlooked in scholarship.

By making the hair covering practices of Orthodox women central, I argue that it represents an external sign of personal dedication to Judaism that empowers these women. This sense of empowerment is especially important for women living in small communities, as they fight to survive in a difficult social environment. Woven into the delicate fabric of American Judaism are threads of the experiences of Orthodoxy in both the American and Jewish world. If one looks closely, deep within the fibers of the fabric are the lives of small town Orthodox Jews. Their stories, especially the voices of the women in these communities, are easily missed. However, their lives contribute to the filaments holding the texture of American Jewry together. By bringing them to the forefront, a new pattern emerges—equally as beautiful but with a slightly different weave.

NOTES

1. Isaac Bashevis Singer, *Yentl the Yeshiva Boy*, translated by Marion Magid and Elizabeth Pollet (New York: Farrar, Straus, and Giroux, 1983).

2. Erich Fromm, *Escape from Freedom* (New York: Holt, 1941); Erich Fromm, *Man for Himself: An Inquiry into the Psychology of Ethics* (New York: Holt, 1947).

3. Rainer Funk, *Erich Fromm: His Life and Ideas, An Illustrated Biography* (New York: Continuum, 2000), 6–31.

4. Funk, *Erich Fromm*, 77.

5. Erich Fromm, *Das jüdische Gesetz: Ein Beitrag zur Soziologie des Diaspora-Judentums* (Weinheim, Germany; Heyne, 1922).

6. See Erich Fromm, *The Sane Society* (New York: Holt, 1955). Fromm also identifies other needs, such as the need to feel related with others, the desire for creativity in developing a meaningful life, the quest for understanding our place in the world, and the desire to feel accomplished.

7. Erich Fromm, *Psychoanalysis and Religion* (New Haven: Yale University Press, 1950), 10–17.

8. Fromm, *Psychoanalysis and Religion*, 94.

9. Fromm, *Psychoanalysis and Religion*, 20.

10. Fromm, *Psychoanalysis and Religion*, 94–95.

11. See Theodor Reik, *Ritual: Psycho-analytic Studies* (New York: Leonard and Virginia Woolf, 1931).

12. Fromm, *Psychoanalysis and Religion*, 108.

13. Fromm, *Psychoanalysis and Religion*, 109–11.

14. Solomon Poll, *The Hasidic Community of Williamsburg: A Study in the Sociology of Religion* (New York: Free Press, 1962), 248.

15. Poll, *Hasidic Community*, 249.

16. Poll, *Hasidic Community*, 250; see Charles Y. Glock, "The Sociology of Religion," in *sociology Today* ed. Robert K. Merton, Leonard Broom, and Leonard S. Cottrell, Jr. (New York: Basic Books 1959), 156. Poll borrows this phrase from Glock.

17. Poll, *Hasidic Community*, 250.

18. Poll, *Hasidic Community*, 250–51.

19. Don Yoder, "Folk Costume," in *Folklore and Folklife: An Introduction*, ed. Richard M. Dorson (Chicago: University of Chicago Press, 1972), 295–324.

20. Yoder, "Folk Costume."

21. Much of the tension that makes this subject electric comes from the idea that American culture has a ritual-destroying, tradition-defying element in which Americans reserve the right to tweak tradition in order to make it "work for them," considering those who affirm tradition to be "Old World."

22. See Renee Kaufman, *Rachel's Daughters: Newly Orthodox Jewish Women* (New Brunswick, NJ: Rutgers University Press, 1991); Lynn Davidman, *Tradition in a Rootless World: Women Turn to Orthodox Judaism* (Berkeley: University of California Press, 1993).

23. Here again I diverge from Fromm, arguing for a multi-layered identity within the everyday context—in this case, situated in Lancaster.

24. Blu Greenberg, *On Women and Judaism: A View from Tradition* (Philadelphia: The Jewish Publication Society of America, 1981).

25. Jewish Orthodox women have worked outside of the home for hundreds of years in order to enable their husbands' scholarship and study. However, their ability to achieve higher paying and higher ranking jobs has been directly impacted by the feminist movement.

26. See Ora Wiskind Elper, *Traditions and Celebrations of the Bat Mitzvah* (New York: Urim, 2003); Sylvia Barack Fishman, *A Breath of Life: Feminism in the American Jewish Community* (Waltham, MA; Brandeis University Press, 1995); Laura Levitt, *Jews and Feminism: The Ambivalent Search for Home* (New York: Psychology Press, 1997); Judith Plaskow, "Jewish Feminist Thought," in *History of Jewish Philosophy*, ed. Daniel H. Frank and Oliver Leaman (New York, Routledge, 1997), 885–895; Judith Plaskow, *Standing Again at Sinai: Judaism from a Feminist Perspective* (New York: Harper, 1991).

27. See Greenberg, *On Women and Judaism*; Jewish Orthodox Feminist Alliance, "Bat Mitzvah" 2011, http://www.jofa.org/social.php/life/batmitzvah (accessed June 28, 2011); Jewish Orthodox Feminist Alliance, "Who We are," 2011, http://www.jofa.org/about.php.who/mission (accessed July 22, 2011); Chana K. Poupko and Devorah Wohlgelernter, "Women's Liberation—An Orthodox Response," in *Tradition* 15, no 4 (Spring, 1976), 45–52.

28. Stephen Stern, *Creative Ethnicity* (Logan: Utah State University Press, 1991).

Epilogue

I recently was sitting in my favorite local coffee shop with an Orthodox friend. A man wearing a white shirt and fedora entered the café and stood at the counter to order. We both stared at him for a moment, not wanting to state the obvious. Finally, I asked her if she knew him. We were both surprised to see an unfamiliar local Orthodox Jew. Through a bit of email exchange and Internet research, we were able, in conjunction with the help of several other Orthodox friends, to sleuth out the identity of the "Mystery Hasid." The man was a local newspaper editor with a fondness for hats, not an Orthodox Jew. I had to laugh. My interviews began with a case of mistaken identity when a coffee shop patron assumed that Vicki was undergoing cancer treatment because of her hair covering. As I neared the close of my investigation, once again the misinterpretation of costuming symbols emerged. This time around, however, I was the one falsely reading symbols.

During a recent service at Degel Israel, I slipped into my favorite seat—two rows back from the Plexiglas portion of the *mechitza* and on the left center aisle. My familiar *Siddur* (prayer book) was nestled safely on the shelf where I had left it the week prior. The spine is cracked from age, and it opens without fail to the *Shema*. Holding it, I remembered back to my first Sabbath service at Degel Israel: I struggled to follow the *Mussaf* service, flipping pages frantically and cursing my rusty Hebrew skills. I was unsure of the social protocol and was, frankly, intimidated. Furthermore, I was fairly certain that although I appreciated tradition, I would not feel any kind of spiritual fulfillment while worshipping at Degel Israel.

My time at Degel Israel has challenged my understanding of feminism. Although I struggle with the embedded patriarchy and division of gender, I find the tradition to be richly spiritual. There have been numerous moments—most notably a rather intense Yom Kippur service—where I am

135

overwhelmed by the beauty of ritual and richness of tradition. The repetition of Hebrew liturgy is a weekly comfort. No matter how stressful my week had been, I know that during my hours at Degel Israel, the chanting of Hebrew, the time for silent prayer, and the sense of community will reroot me as I head into the next work week. I have experienced the Sabbath in ways which had previously been unknown to me.

Moreover, the congregation has come to mean something special to me. The familiar smell of the building, trekking in from the alley parking lot with the others who drive on the Sabbath, the warm "Good Shabbos!" greetings, and even the pickled herring are now familiar. Initially I did not expect to make friends within the congregation, and I understood that as an outsider I would likely be viewed skeptically. It took time to find my place within Degel Israel, but I am grateful that they have allowed me into their lives. In the beginning, I was aware that I was carefully watched and maybe even at times judged. However, after a spinal injury took me out of commission for an entire summer, it was the women of Degel Israel who came to my home, bringing food, smiles, and kind words. They phoned me frequently to check in on my health, offered to drive me to doctor's appointments, and worried about the impact that the injury and subsequent surgery would have on my family, career, and research. Suddenly I was no longer an outsider. They accepted me, bad back and all, into their lives, and for this, I am eternally grateful.

At the conclusion of this study, I recognize that my social connections will remain with the women who have become such special friends. Religiously, though, I will seek my home in a more liberal congregation. However, I will continue to be a voice and advocate for tradition, the importance of which Degel Israel has taught me. Financially I will also continue to do my best to support the fundraising efforts of the synagogue. I understand, more than ever before, the financial hardship they experience as such a small community.

During a recent conversation with Rosemary, one of the women interviewed in chapter five, she reflected, "I think you may have made me realize that I might be a little bit feminist, but I still hate that word." I smiled and responded, "And I think that you have made me realize that even though I consider myself an adamant feminist, I still really love tradition." We both nodded in understanding. We are, after all, more alike than we are different.

Glossary

Ashkenazic Jews	Lit. from the region of Germany and northern France called "Ashkenaz" during the Middle Ages; Jews with German and Eastern European roots.
Ba'alot teshuva	[Hebrew] Jews who recommit themselves to Judaism and begin to live a religiously observant lifestyle; those who are newly observant.
Basari	[Hebrew] Pertaining to foods that fall under the meat category under kosher dietary laws; also known as *fleischig* in Yiddish.
Bimah	[Hebrew] The platform area in the synagogue; the place from where scripture is read.
Chavrusa	[Aramaic] Lit. friend or companion; a study pairing that is one of the unique features of Yeshiva-style learning where the partners learn, discuss, and debate religious texts.
Daven	[Yiddish] to pray; the Yiddish has been Anglicized to make the active form davening.
Eruv (pl. eruvin)	[Hebrew] A ritual enclosure or fence around a home or community that allows for the carrying of objects during the Sabbath.
Fleischig	[Yiddish] Pertaining to foods that fall under the meat category in kosher dietary laws; also known as *basari* in Hebrew.

Frum	[Yiddish] from the German "fromm," meaning pious; pertaining to those who are religiously devout or observant.
Halakha	[Hebrew] The collective body of Jewish law; can also reference individual Jewish laws.
Halakhic	[Hebrew] Pertaining to Jewish legal codes; in accordance with *halakha*.
Halavi	[Hebrew] Pertaining to foods that fall under the dairy category under kosher dietary laws; also known as *milchig* in Hebrew.
Judenhut	[German] Lit. a Jew-hat; a cone-shaped hat that Jews were forced to wear in Medieval Europe to identify them when outside of the ghetto.
Kasher	[Hebrew/Yiddish] The act of rendering something kosher; the Yiddish has been Anglicized to make the active form kashering.
Kashrut	[Hebrew/Yiddish] The set of Jewish dietary laws that are in accordance with *halakha*; laws determining which foods are permitted and forbidden in order for something to be considered kosher.
Kiddush	[Hebrew] The blessing said over wine during the Sabbath and Jewish holidays.
Kippah (pl. kippot)	[Hebrew] Cap, the traditionally male Jewish skullcap; the Anglicized plural is sometimes rendered kippahs; also known as *yarmulke* in Yiddish.
Klal Yisrael	[Hebrew] The collective responsibility for the Jewish community.
Mechitza	[Hebrew] A partition that separates men and women in the sanctuary of a synagogue.
Mikveh (pl. mikvot)	[Hebrew] The bath used for ritual immersion; the ritual bath used to remove or nullify ritual impurities.
Milchig	[Yiddish] Pertaining to foods that fall under the dairy category under kosher dietary laws; also known as *halavi* in Hebrew.
Minhag	[Hebrew] Lit. for "driving" (2 Kings 9:20); understood in modern Jewish tradition as a custom representing a local cultural norm.

Minyan (pl. minyanim)	[Hebrew] The quorum of ten men required for certain religious events and rituals.
Mitzvah (pl. mitzvot)	[Hebrew] A commandment, understood to be of divine origin.
Negel vasser	[Yiddish] Lit. "nail water;" ritual hand washing; also known as *netilat yadayim* in Hebrew.
Netilat yadayim	[Hebrew] Ritual hand washing; also known as *negel vasser* in Yiddish.
Niddah	[Hebrew] A woman who is considered ritually impure during the time of menstruation; pertaining to the laws of family or sexual purity.
Olam haba	[Hebrew] Jewish eschatological phrase referring to the time after the Messiah.
Parve	[Yiddish] Those foods which fall under the neutral category of kosher dietary laws, including fish, fruits, vegetables, and spices.
Payos	[Yiddish] Sidelocks or sidecurls worn by Jewish men; also known as *payot* in Hebrew.
Payot	[Hebrew] Sidelocks or sidecurls worn by Jewish men; also known as *payos* in Yiddish.
Rosh Chodesh	[Hebrew] The new Jewish month; begins with the appearance of the new moon; associated with women's gatherings.
Shabbat	[Hebrew] The Jewish Sabbath; also known as *Shabbos* in Yiddish.
Shabbos	[Yiddish] The Jewish Sabbath; also known as *Shabbat* in Hebrew.
Sephardic Jews	[Hebrew] Jews with Spanish and north-African roots.
Shadchan (pl. shadchanim)	[Hebrew] Professional Orthodox matchmaker; the plural is often Anglicized to Schadchans.
Sheitel (pl. sheiteln,)	[Yiddish] A wig worn in order to cover the hair; the plural is often Anglicized to sheitels.
Shidduchim	[Hebrew, pl]. Matches made for marriage within the Orthodox community; typically made by a *Shadchan*.

Shpitzel (pl. shpitzeln)	[Yiddish] A head covering worn by some Hasidic women that has a braid of hair across the front and is covered by a *tichel*; the plural is often Anglicized to schpitzels.
Shomer shabbos	[Yiddish] Those who are strictly observant of the Sabbath laws, refusing to drive, carry items, write, or engage in any other form of work.
Shtreimel (pl. shtreimlech)	[Yiddish] Fur hats worn by Hasidic men; the plural is often Anglicized to shtreimels.
Shul	[Yiddish] Lit. School; Yiddish for synagogue.
Siddur (pl. Siddurim)	[Hebrew] A Jewish prayer book, including the set order of daily prayers, Sabbath service, and other Jewish services.
Siman nisuin	[Hebrew] A sign of marriage.
Snood	[English] A close-fitting hood that encases the hair in a small sack.
Sukkah	[Hebrew] A walled structure covered with branches in which to eat, celebrate, and entertain guests during the Jewish holiday of Sukkot.
Tallis (pl. tallisim)	[Yiddish] The prayer shawl worn over the shoulders or head; the plural is often Anglicized to tallises.
Tallit (pl. tallitot)	[Hebrew] The prayer shawl worn over the shoulders or head.
Tefillin	[Hebrew] The leather cases enclosing scripture written on parchment that are bound to the forehead and left arm; also known as phylacteries from the Greek.
Tichel (pl. ticheln)	[Yiddish] A headscarf worn over the hair; the plural is typically Anglicized to tichels.
Tzitzit	[Hebrew] The knotted ritual fringes worn by observant Jews.
Tznius	[Yiddish] Modesty and humility; pertaining to conduct between the sexes; referring to dressing modestly; also known as *tzniut* in Hebrew.
Tzniusdik	[Yiddish] Of or pertaining to being in a state of modesty.

Tzniut	[Hebrew] Modesty and humility; pertaining to conduct between the sexes; referring to dressing modestly; also known as *tznius* in Yiddish.
Yarmulke (pl. yarmulkes)	[Yiddish] The traditionally male Jewish skullcap; also known as *kippah* in Hebrew.
Yeshiva (pl. yeshivot)	[Hebrew/Yiddish] A Jewish educational institution or school that focuses on the daily study of traditional religious texts, particularly the Talmud and Torah.
Yiddishkeit	[Yiddish] Lit. Jewishness; pertaining to the Jewish way of life; referring to a measurement of how observant or culturally Jewish a person is.

Bibliography

Adler, Cyrus. 1900. *American Jewish Yearbook: September 25, 1900 to September 13, 1901.* Philadelphia: Jewish Publication Society of America.

Adler, Rachel. 1972. "The Jew Who Wasn't There: Halakhah and the Jewish Woman." *Davka* (Summer 1972): 7–13.

Agar, Michael. 1996. *The Professional Stranger: An Informal Introduction to Ethnography.* New York: Emerald Group.

Alpert, Rebecca, and Jacob Staub. 2000. *Exploring Judaism: A Reconstructionist Approach.* NewYork: The Reconstructionist Press.

Ament, Jonathon. 2005. *American Jewish Religious Denominations.* New York: National Jewish Population Survey.

America's Next Top Model. Season 14, episode 2. First broadcast March 17, 2010 by The CW Network. Produced by Tyra Banks, Ken Mok, and Daniel Soiseth.

Amphlett, Hilda. 2003. *Hats: A History of Fashion in Headwear.* New York: Dover Publications.

Asher-Greve, Julia M. 1985. *Frauen in Altsumerischer Zeit.* Berlin: Undena.

The Association of Religion Data Archives. 2010a. "Lancaster County, Pennsylvania." Accessed December 28. http://www.thearda.com/mapsReports/reports/counties/42071_2000 .asp.

———. 2010b. "The United States, General." Accessed December 28. http://www.thearda .com/internationalData/countries/Country_234_1.asp.

Baizerman, Suzanne. 1992. "The Jewish *kippah sruga* and the Social Construction of Gender in Israel." In *Dress and Gender: Making and Meaning,* edited by Ruth Barnes and Joanne B. Eicher, 92-105. New York: Berg Publishers, 1992.

Baskin, Judith. 1991. "Jewish Women in the Middle Ages." In *Jewish Women in Historical Perspective,* edited by Judith R. Baskin, 101–27. Detroit: Wayne State University Press.

Benesch, Hellmuth. 1995. "Neo-Psychoanalyse." In *Enzyklopädisches Wörterbuch Klinische Psychologie und Psychotherapie,* edited by Hellmuth Benesch, 550–70. Weinheim, Germany: Beltz.

Berg, Charles. 1951. *The Unconscious Significance of Hair.* London: George Allen and Unwin.

Brener, David. 1979. *The Jews of Lancaster, Pennsylvania: A Story with Two Beginnings.* Lancaster, PA: Congregation Shaarai Shomayim.

Bronner, Leila Leah. 1993. "From Veil to Wig: Jewish Women's Hair Covering." *Judaism: A Quarterly Journal of Jewish Life and Thought* (Fall 1993): 465–77.

Buhle, Mari Jo. 2000. *Feminism and Its Discontents: A Century of Struggle with Psychoanalysis.* Cambridge, MA: Harvard University Press.

Byrd, Ayana. 2002. *Hair Story: Untangling the Roots of Black Hair in America*. New York: St. Martin's Press.

Carrell, Barbara Goldman. 1999. "Hasidic Women's Head Coverings." In *Religion, Dress and the Body*, edited by Linda B. Arthur, 163–80. Oxford, UK: Oxford University Press.

Chodorow, Nancy J. 1991. *Feminism and Psychoanalytic Theory*. New Haven: Yale University Press.

Clark, Fiona. 1984. *Hats*. New York: Quite Specific Media Group.

Crane, Diana. 2000. *Fashion and Its Social Agendas: Class, Gender, and Identity in Clothing*. Chicago: University of Chicago Press.

Croom, Alexandra. 2010. *Roman Clothing and Fashion*. New York: Amberly.

Cunningham, Michael and Craig Marberry. 2000. *Crowns: Portraits of Black Women in Church Hats*. Ann Arbor: University of Michigan Press.

Da Silva, Filipe Carreira. 2007. *G. H. Mead: A Critical Introduction*. New York: Polity.

Davidman, Lynn. 1993. *Tradition in a Rootless World: Women Turn to Orthodox Judaism*. Berkley: University of California Press.

Davis, Eli and Elise Davis. 1983. *Hats and Caps of the Jews*. Jerusalem: Masada.

Davis, Moshe. 1963. *The Emergence of Conservative Judaism*. Philadelphia: Jewish Publication Society of America.

Deleuze, Gilles and Felix Guattari. 1983. *Anti-Oedipus: Capitalism and Schizophrenia*. Minneapolis: University of Minnesota Press.

Diamond, Etan. 2000. *And I Will Dwell in Their Midst: Orthodox Jews in Suburbia*. Chapel Hill: University of North Carolina Press, 5.

Diner, Hasia. 2006. *The Jews of the United States, 1654–2000*. Berkeley: University of California Press.

DuBois, W. E. B. 1994. *The Souls of Black Folk*. New York: Gramercy Books.

Dundes, Alan. 1987. *Parsing Through Customs: Essays by a Freudian Folklorist*. Madison: University of Wisconsin Press.

Elper, Ora Wiskind. 2003. *Traditions and Celebrations of the Bat Mitzvah*. New York: Urim.

Falk, Pesach Eliyahu. 1998. *Modesty: An Adornment for Life: Halachos and Attitudes Concerning Tznius of Dress and Conduct*. New York: Philipp Feldheim.

———. 2002. *Sheitels: A Halachic Guide to Present-Day Sheitels*. Jerusalem: Bnos Melochim.

Fishman, Sylvia Barack. 1995. *A Breath of Life: Feminism in the American Jewish Community*. Waltham, MA: Brandeis University Press.

Frankel, Elle. 1997. *Five Books of Miriam: A Woman's Commentary on the Torah*. New York: HarperOne.

Fromm, Erich. 1922. *Das jüdische Gesetz: Ein Beitrag zur Soziologie des Diaspora-Judentums*. Weinheim, Germany: Heyne.

———. 1990. *Die Entdeckung des gesellschaftlichen Unbewussten: Zur Neubestimmung der Psychoanalyse*. Weinheim, Germany: Beltz.

———. 1941. *Escape from Freedom*. New York: Holt.

———. 1947. *Man for Himself: An Inquiry into the Psychology of Ethics*. New York: Holt.

———. 1950. *Psychoanalysis and Religion*. New Haven: Yale University Press.

———. 1955. *The Sane Society*. New York: Holt.

Funk, Rainer. 2000. *Erich Fromm: His Life and Ideas, An Illustrated Biography*. New York: Continuum.

Gillman, Neil. 1993. *Conservative Judaism: The New Century*. New York: Behrman.

Ginsburg, Madeline. 1990. *The Hat: Trends and Traditions*. New York: Barrons.

Glock, Charles Y. 1959. "The Sociology of Religion." In *Sociology Today*, edited by Robert K. Merton, Leonard Broom, and Leonard S. Cottrell, Jr. New York: Basic Books.

Goffman, Erving. 1961. *Asylums: Essays on the Social Situation of Mental Patients and other Inmates*. New York: Anchor.

———. 1965. "Identity Kits." In *Dress, Adornment and the Social Orders*, edited by M. Roach and J. Eicher, 246–47. New York: John Wiley and Sons.

———. 1959. *The Presentation of Self in Everyday Life*. New York: Anchor.

Goldstein, Elyse M. 2008. *The Women's Torah Commentary*. New York: Jewish Lights Publishing.

Gordon, Albert. 1959. *Jews in Suburbia*. Boston: Beacon Press.

Greenberg, Blu. 1981. *On Women and Judaism: A View from Tradition*. Philadelphia: The Jewish Publication Society of America.

Griebel, Helen Bradley. 1995. "The African American Woman's Headwrap: Unwinding the Symbols." In *Dress and Identity*, edited by Mary Ellen Roach-Higgins, Joanne B. Eicher, and Kim K. P. Johnson, 445–60. New York: Capital Cities Media.

Guimón, José. 2004. *Relational Mental Health: Beyond Evidence-Based Interventions*. New York: Springer.

Gurock, Jeffrey S. 2009. *Orthodox Jews in America*. Bloomington: Indiana University Press.

Heilman, Samuel. 1999. *Defenders of the Faith: Inside Ultra-Orthodox Jewry*. Berkeley: University of California Press.

———. 2006. *Sliding to the Right: The Contest for the Future of American Jewish Orthodoxy*. Berkeley: University of California Press.

Heilman, Samuel and Steven Cohen. 1999. *Cosmopolitans and Parochials: Modern Orthodox Jews in America*. Chicago: University of Chicago Press.

Heschel, Abraham Joshua. 2005. *The Sabbath*, New York: Farrar Straus Giroux.

Heschel, Susannah. 1987. *On Begin a Jewish Feminist*. New York: Schocken.

Hyman, Paula E. 1995. *Gender and Assimilation in Modern Jewish History: The Roles and Representation of Women*. Seattle: University of Washington Press.

Jacobs, Meredith. 2007. *The Modern Jewish Mom's Guide to Shabbat; Connect and Celebrate—Bring Your Family Together with the Friday Night Meal*. New York: Harper Books.

Jaffe, Azriela. 2005. *What Do You Mean, You Can't Eat in My Home?: A Guide to How Newly Observant Jews and Their Less Observant Relatives Can Still Get Along*. New York: Schocken.

The Jewish Federations of North America. 2011. "National Jewish Population Survey: Orthodox Jews." Accessed June 22. http://www.jewishfederations.org/local_includes/downloads/4983.pdf.

Jewish Orthodox Feminist Alliance. 2011a. "Bat Mitzvah." Accessed June 28. http://www.jofa.org/social.php/life/batmitzvah.

———. 2011b. "Who We Are." Accessed July 22. http://www.jofa.org/about.php.who/mission.

Jones, Stephen. 2009. *Hats: An Anthology*. London: V & A Publishing.

Joselit, Jenna Weissman. 2002. *The Wonders of America: Reinventing Jewish Culture 1880–1950*. New York: Picado.

Kaplan, Dana Evan. 2003. *American Reform Judaism: An Introduction*. New Brunswick, NJ: Rutgers University Press.

Kaufman, Renee. 1991. *Rachel's Daughters: Newly Orthodox Jewish Women*. New Brunswick, NJ: Rutgers University Press.

Kelley, Dean M. 1996. *Why Conservative Churches are Growing: A Study in Sociology of Religion*. Macon, GA: Mercer University Press.

Kugelmass, Jack. 1996. *The Miracle of Intervale Avenue: The Story of a Jewish Congregation in the South Bronx*. New York: Columbia University Press.

Landau, David. 1992. *Piety and Power: The World of Jewish Fundamentalism*. New York: Hill and Wang.

Leach, E. R. 1958. "Magical Hair." *The Journal of the Royal Anthropological Institute of Great Britain and Ireland* 88 (July–December): 147–64.

Levinger, Lee J. 1952. "The Disappearing Small-Town Jew." *Commentary* 14 (July–December): 1961–62.

Levitt, Laura. 1997. *Jews and Feminism: The Ambivalent Search for Home*. New York: Psychology Press.

Liebow, Elliot. 1967. *Tally's Corner: A Study of Negro Streetcorner Men*. Lanham, MD: Rowman and Littlefield.

———. 1995. *Tell Them Who I Am: The Lives of Homeless Women*. New York: Penguin.

Lynd, Robert S. and Helen Merrell Lynd. 1959. *Middletown: A Study in Modern American Culture*. New York: Harcourt Brace Javanovich.

Maier, Johann. 1972. *Geschichte der jüdischen Religion: Von der Zeit Alexander des Grossen bis zur Aufklärung mit einem Ausblick of das 19./20. Jahrhundert* Frankfurt: De Gruyter.

McCracken, Grant. 1995. *Big Hair: A Journey into the Transformation of Self.* Woodstock, NY: Overlook Press.

McDowell, Colin. 1992. *Hats: Status, Style, and Glamour.* New York: Rizzoli.

Mead, George Herbert. 1934. *Mind, Self, and Society.* Chicago: University of Chicago Press.

———. 1938. *The Philosophy of the Act.* Chicago: University of Chicago Press.

Meyers, Carol and Toni Craven, Ross Shephard Kraemer. 2001. *Women in Scripture: A Dictionary of Named and Unnamed Women in the Bible, the Apocrypha/Deuterocanonical Books, and the New Testament.* New York: Eerdmans.

Mintz, Jerome. 1998. *Hasidic People: A Place in the New World.* Cambridge, MA: Harvard University Press.

Mitchell, Juliet and Sangay Mishra, 1974. *Psychoanalysis and Feminism: A Radical Reassessment of Freudian Psychoanalysis.* New York: Basic Books.

National Vital Statistics Report. 2011. "Births." Accessed July 19. http://www.cdc.gov/nchs/data/nvsr/nvsr59/nvsr59_03.pdf.

Nemet-Nejat, Karen Rhea. 2001. *Daily Life in Ancient Mesopotamia.* New York: Baker.

Newsom, Carol A. and Sharon H. Ringe. 1998. *Women's Bible Commentary.* New York: Westminster.

Obeyesekere, Gananath. 1984. *Medusa's Hair: An Essay on Personal Symbols and Religious Experience.* Chicago: University of Chicago Press.

Olson, Kelly. 2008. *Dress and the Roman Woman: Self Presentation and Society.* New York: Routledge.

Philips, Adam. 1996. *On Flirtation.* Cambridge, MA: Harvard University Press.

Plaskow, Judith. 1997. "Jewish Feminist Thought." In *History of Jewish Philosophy,* edited by Daniel H. Frank and Oliver Leaman, 885–95. New York: Routledge.

———. 1991. *Standing Again at Sinai: Judaism from a Feminist Perspective.* New York: Harper.

Pointon, Marcia. 2009. "Materializing Mourning: Hair, Jewellery, and the Body." In *Fashion: Critical and Primary Sources: The Nineteenth Century,* edited by Peter McNeil, 345–58. Oxford, UK: Berg.

Poll, Solomon. 1962. *The Hasidic Community of Williamsburg: A Study in the Sociology of Religion.* New York: Free Press.

Poupko, Chana K. and Devorah Wohlgelernter. 1976. "Women's Liberation—An Orthodox Response." *Tradition* 15, no. 4 (Spring): 45–52.

Prince, Althea. 2010. *The Politics of Black Women's Hair.* New York: Idiomatic.

Probert, Christina. 1981. *Hats in Vogue since 1910.* New York: Abbeville Press.

Redfield, Robert, Robert Linton, and Melville Herskovits. 1936. "Memorandum for the Study of Acculturation." *American Anthropologist* 38: 149–52.

Reik, Theodor. 1931. *Ritual: Psycho-analytic Studies.* New York: Leonard and Virginia Woolf.

Reynolds, Margaret. 2001. *Plain Women: Gender and Ritual in the Old Order River Brethren.* University Park: Pennsylvania State University Press.

Rieger, Miriam. 2004. *The American Jewish Elderly.* New York: National Jewish Population Survey.

Robinson, Fred Miller. 1993. *The Man in the Bowler Hat: Its History and Iconography.* Chapel Hill: University of North Carolina Press.

Rose, Peter. 1977. *Strangers in Their Midst: Small-Town Jews and Their Neighbors.* New York: Richwood Publishing.

Ross, Tamar. 2004. *Expanding the Palace of Torah: Orthodoxy and Feminism.* Waltham, MA: Brandeis University Press.

Rubins, Alfred, 1973. *A History of Jewish Costumes.* New York: Crown, 8–11.

Ruttenberg, Danya, editor. 2001. *Yentl's Revenge: The Next Wave of Jewish Feminism.* New York: Seal Press.

Sackett, Shaya. 2011. "The Lancaster Yeshiva Center." Accessed June 25. http://www.lancasteryeshiva.com/.

Sarna, Jonathan D. 2005. *American Judaism: A History.* New Haven: Yale University Press.

Schreiber, Lynne. 2006. *Hide and Seek: Jewish Women and Hair Covering.* New York: Urim Publications.

Sefer Dat Yehudit K'hilkhata. 1973. Jerusalem: The Committee for the Preservation of Modesty.

Sherrow, Victoria. 2006. *Encyclopedia of Hair: A Cultural History.* Westport, CT: Greenwood.

Sheskin, Ira M. 2004. *Geographical Differences Among American Jews.* New York: National Jewish Population Survey.

———. 2011. "Recent Trends in Jewish Demographics and Their Impact on the Jewish Media—June 2011." Accessed June 20. http://www.jewishdatabank.org/Reports/Recent-Trends_Sheskin_2011.pdf.

Sheskin, Ira M. and Arnold Dashefsky. 2010. *Jewish Population in the United States, 2010.* Storrs, CT: Jewish Data Bank and the Jewish Federations of North America.

Showstack, Gerald Lee. 1988. *Suburban Communities: The Jewishness of American Reform Jews.* New York: Scholars Press.

Simon, Diane. 2001. *Hair: Public, Political, Extremely Personal.* New York: St. Martin's Press.

Singer, Isaac Bashevis. 1983. *Yentl the Yeshiva Boy.* Translated by Marion Magid and Elizabeth Pollet. New York: Farrar, Straus and Giroux.

Sklare, Marshall. 1967. *Jewish Identity on the Suburban Frontier: A Study of Group Survival in the Open Society.* Chicago: University of Chicago Press.

Steinberg, Neil. 2004. *Hatless Jack: The President, the Fedora, and the History of American Style.* New York: Plume.

Stern, Lise. 2004. *How to Keep Kosher: A Comprehensive Guide to Understanding Jewish Dietary Laws.* New York: William Morrow.

Stern, Stephen. 1991. *Creative Ethnicity.* Logan: Utah State University Press.

United Jewish Communities. 2011. "Jews in Small Communities." Accessed June 23. http://www.jewishfederations.org/local_includes/downloads/5542.pdf.

———. 2004. "National Jewish Population Survey 2000–01—Orthodox Jews: A United Jewish Communities Presentation of Findings." Accessed June 24. http://www.jewishdatabank.org/Archive/NJPS2000_Orthodox_Jews.pdf.

The US Census Bureau. 2011a. "Lancaster (city), Pennsylvania." Accessed January 6. http://quickfacts.census.gov/qfd/states/42/4241216.html.

———. 2011b. "Lancaster County, Pennsylvania." Accessed January 6. http://quickfacts.census.gov/qfd/states/42/42071.html.

———. 2011c. "Lancaster County, Pennsylvania—Educational Attainment." Accessed May 16. http://factfinder.census.gov/servlet/STTable?_bm=y&-geo_id=05000US42071&-qr_name=ACS_2009_5YR_G00_S1501&-ds_name=ACS_2009_5YR_G00_&-redoLog=false.

Weissbach, Lee Shai. 2005. *Jewish Life in Small-Town America: A History.* New Haven: Yale University Press.

Weitz, Rose. 2004. *Rapunzel's Daughters: What Women's Hair Tells Us About Women's Lives.* New York: Farrar, Straus and Giroux.

Wenger, Etienne. 1998. *Communities of Practice: Learning, Meaning, and Identity.* Cambridge, UK: Cambridge University Press.

———. 2011. "Communities of Practice." Accessed June 20. http://www.ewenger.com/theory/
.

Wenger, Etienne and Jean Lave. 1990. *Situated Learning: Legitimate Peripheral Participation.* Cambridge, UK: Cambridge University Press.

Wertheimer, Jack. 2011. "Low Fertility and High Intermarriage are Pushing American Jewry Toward Extinction." Accessed July 19. http://www.aish.com/jw/s/48899452.html.

Wylen, Stephen M. 2000. *Settings of Silver: An Introduction to Judaism.* New York: Paulist Press.

Yoder, Don. 1972. "Folk Costume." In *Folklore and Folklife: An Introduction*, ed. Richard M. Dorson, 295–324. Chicago: University of Chicago Press.

Index

About the Author

Amy K. Milligan currently teaches women and gender studies at Elizabeth-town College. Her research concentrates on the overlap of gender and sexuality with religion. In particular, she is interested in the literal embodiment of religious faith or group affiliation, with particular attention given to evolutions of material culture. Her current research concentrates on the use of yarmulkes, tattoos, and other externalizations of identity by the LGBTQ community.

CPSIA information can be obtained at www.ICGtesting.com
Printed in the USA
BVOW07*0439160914

366930BV00003B/10/P

9 780739 183656